Table of Contents

Chapter 5. Low Fiber Recipes

Chapter 6. High Fiber Recipes

Breakfast

Conclusion

Introduction

In older times, people used to have full grains, fibers and lots of vegetables. Thus, digestive diseases were rare and often unheard of. Taken into account the huge change in the consumption patterns of people around the globe in the last century, such digestive diseases have become commonplace. People have adopted diets that are high in fat and sugar content. Such diets are devoid of essential nutrients and most importantly, the fibers that help in easy digestion and effective absorption of the nutrients.

Also, people do not take care of the liquid intake in the body and consume sodas and other drinks instead of plain replenishing water. A combination of fiber deficient diet along with lack of water content in the body gives rise to conditions of constipation. People experience difficulty in passing on the stool, which gets stuck in the colon region giving rise to condition of Diverticulosis which later advances to a severe stage, called Diverticulitis.

The vegetarians are the least affected by the disease since their diet is laden with fiber coming from grains, fruits and vegetables. The non-vegetarians are at greater risk of contracting Diverticulitis. Reports have it that the meat-eating western countries like America and the European nations have greater cases of the disease than the Asian countries where several of them have a vegetarian diet as their staple food. Africans have been least affected by the disease owing to their not so rich in fat diet.

Sedentary lifestyles and lack of exercise along with proper conditioning of the body adds to the worsening of the condition. The disease is very difficult to diagnose in absence of any specific symptoms. It is often neglected in the earlier stages in lieu of ordinary digestive ailments and is not given much attention. The disease is progressive in nature and the situation deteriorates in absence of proper attentiveness.

Diverticulitis is a chronic digestive disease which involves the development of sacs or pouches in the bowel wall. These pouches are typically known as diverticula that appear on the sides of the longitudinal muscle surrounding the colon wall. This disease typically occurs in the colon or the large intestines. However, small intestines could also be affected by it.

Diverticulitis is the inflammation of one of these several diverticula. The inflammation can also be accompanied with acute infection that is often detrimental to health. Diverticulitis in its milder forms is known as Diverticulosis which is a commonly known medical condition. The most common symptoms a person with Diverticulitis shows is the excessive and continued pain in the lower abdominal region accompanied by fever and dizziness. The patient may also see sizeable increase in the white blood cell count.

The most common reason for development of the disease is assumed to be a fiber deficient diet. The disease is also associated with old age as the bowel system gets weaker as a person ages. Reports have it that almost all people above the age of 70 have been affected by Diverticulitis.

Chapter 1. What is diverticulitis

Mild cases of diverticulitis are treated with antibiotics but those suffering from severe diverticulitis may have to rest eating by mouth and may adopt a special type of diet until the bleeding and pain subside. The Diverticulitis Diet is a highly recommended diet that can help alleviate acute diverticulitis. Although this diet is supposed to be short-term, it can bring about huge relief among individuals who suffer from diverticulitis. Moreover, it can also be used by people who have a sensitive digestive system.

While the Diverticulitis Diet is designed for people who suffer from diverticulitis, people who suffer from other digestive distress can benefit from the Diverticulitis diet. Moreover, normal healthy individuals who also want to give their digestive tract enough rest can benefit from this diet.

Phases of the Diverculitis Diet

Phase 1: Clear Fluids (During A Flare)

While going through an active flare, your symptoms can become extreme. Due to this it's smart for you to give your bowel a period of rest. As you can imagine the best way to do this is by sticking to a clear fluid diet. This will aid in your recovery as your body may outright reject solid foods.

It is vital to note that the clear fluid stage of the diet is NOT intended to be a long-term diet. In fact, the general expectation is that you remain in this stage for no more than a couple of days.

Please Note:

Restricting yourself to a clear fluid diet for an excessive amount of time may cause you to feel light-headed, weak, hungry, and fatigued. You can also experience muscle wasting, excessive weight loss, and depletion of vitamins and minerals.

This occurs due to the fact that it's incredibly difficult to meet the body's daily caloric requirements for fat, protein, and carbohydrates through a clear fluid diet. The average person will need to provide their body with at least 200 grams of carbohydrates to have enough energy to go through the day. If you struggle with low blood sugar, diabetes, or other blood sugar challenges, you may want to monitor your blood sugar levels during this stage.

As the name implies, this phase is composed of clear liquids. These include green tea, fresh fruit juice, clear broth, and gelatin dessert. The clear liquid diet provides the body with salt, liquids, and enough nutrients to function temporarily, generally for a few days, until you can eat normal food.

Phase 2: Low-Residue/Low Fiber Diet (Immediately After A Controlled Flare)

A low-residue (or low-fiber) diet acts as the reintroduction phase, after your flare-up symptoms have mostly passed but before your body is ready for high-fiber or high residue foods.

Phase 3: High Fiber Meals (Daily Life/ Preventing Future Flares)

This final stage in the diverticulitis diet is the High Fiber diet. This stage is used to maintain a balanced diet while preventing a future flare. It is basically your general day to day eating routine, and generally takes up the majority of your diverticulitis eating plan.

It is important to note, however, that you do not want to jump directly from a significantly low fiber diet (such as a clear fluid diet) directly to a high fiber diet, as this will do more harm to your colon than good. It is always best to ease into any stage of the plan that requires an increase in your fiber intake. Aim to increase your fiber intake by 2 to 4 grams per week until you reach the recommended amount for your age and biology. Bear in mind that as you increase your fiber, you also need to increase your water intake to help move the fiber through your intestinal tract.

Chapter 2. Causes and Symptoms

It is unclear why diverticula forms, and many experts have varying opinions on the subject. For some, strains or muscle spasms, especially during bowel movements, is the key reason for pressure buildup in the colon, which pushes against the inner lining. Formerly, many experts believed that inadequate consumption of fiber, which can be found in vegetables and fruits, legumes, and grains, can result in diverticulosis. However, recent inquiries into the subject are yet to reveal any clear relationship between diverticula and the consumption of fiber-rich foods.

Another potential theory is that, although unsure of the original triggers of diverticulitis, infection tends to begin as a result of the bacteria content in stools that are pushed into the diverticula. A different theory posits that the walls of the diverticula are subject to erosions from constant and increased pressure levels in the walls of the colon.

Symptoms of Diverticulitis

Although diverticulitis isn't known to result in bothersome symptoms, people tend to report any of the following conditions:

- Constipation
- Mild abdominal cramps
- Tenderness over the affected area
- Bloating or swelling

Bear in mind that presenting with one or more of the symptoms mentioned above isn't necessarily an indication that you suffer from diverticulosis. These symptoms are quite common and present in several gastrointestinal disorders ranging from stomach ulcers to inflammatory bowel diseases to irritable bowel syndrome to gallstones to celiac disease to appendicitis.

How Diverticulitis Is Diagnosed

Since symptoms of diverticulitis do not readily present in many people, the condition is usually discovered when the patient is being screened for polyps or evaluated for other conditions. Gastroenterologists can easily locate and reveal diverticula in the colon using a procedure that requires a tiny camera attached to the end of a lighted, flexible tube that is inserted into the rectum.

Another procedure that can be used is sigmoidoscopy in which a short tube is used to probe the lower areas of the colon and the rectum alone. For colonoscopy procedures, a longer tube is used and the whole colon is examined. However, the discovery of diverticulosis isn't limited to gastrointestinal procedures alone, and can also be discovered via imaging tests such as barium x-rays and computer tomography (CT) scan.

How Is Diverticulitis Treated?

When diverticula develops on the colon, they don't tend to occur on their own. For most patients, the symptoms never present and no treatments are necessary. However, when the condition is accompanied by symptoms, such as constipation, bloating, bleeding, and abdominal pain, your doctor could place you on a diet with high fiber content. The choice of diet is meant to soften stools and make them easier to pass. According to daily requirements, it's advised that we consume about 20 to 35 grams of fibre, even though many people only ever consume about half of the said amount daily.

The easiest method of improving fiber intake is to consume more grains, vegetables, and fruits. Some examples of foods with high, healthy fiber content include lima beans, broccoli, apples, squash, kidney beans, pears, and baked beans. Alternatively, your doctor could recommend fiber supplements such as polycarbophil, methylcellulose, or psyllium. These products tend to come in different forms like wafers, powders, or pills. Supplemental fiber products work like high-fiber foods, helping to soften and bulk up stool, making bowel movements easier and less strenuous. Your doctor could also prescribe some medication to reduce the level of colon spasms, which can result in discomfort and abdominal cramping.

Chapter 3. How to Improve Gut Flora

The human body is comprised of over 40 trillion bacteria that has multiple purposes, a number which reside in your intestines. The good bacteria as a collective are referred to as the gut microbiota or gut flora, and they play an extremely vital part in maintaining your overall health. The bad bacteria that form, on the other hand, contributes to many different diseases.

Due to this it is vital that you take care of your gut to ensure that most the bacteria residing in your body is good bacteria. As you may have already guessed, the food you consume plays a significant role in the type of bacteria that grow inside you.

Let's explore a few simple ways you can improve your gut flora:

- Maintaining Bacterial Balance

One of the symptoms that are very common in diverticulitis patients is the intestinal bacterial overgrowth. That is too much development of harmful bacteria which leads to inflammation and damage to the entire system and makes all digestion less effective. Rifaximin is a drug that has been shown to affect this issue in a positive way by returning the bacterial balance to a more normal level. There are also simple foods that will do this as well, including some specialty yogurts.

- Take Related Supplements

A person suffering from diverticulitis may be able to find some significant relief by taking probiotic supplements. In combination with other treatments the probiotic nutrients can give a person a whole new lease on life. There are some great food choices that already include probiotics in them for example eating foods with kefir, kimchi or kombucha in them will naturally help reduce the effects of diverticulitis.

Adding a supplement like Prescript Assist or VSL#3 is not a bad idea no matter where your health is currently at because it will improve your digestion and allow you to feel healthier each day.

- Probiotics

It is important to make sure probiotics are in your diet. Probiotics will add healthy bacteria to the digestive system and make the colon work smoother and more efficiently which will allow for less development of Diverticular disease. Probiotics enhance the ability of the body to take the nutrients from food, breakdown lactose and even help improve the immune system of the body. Low fat yogurt or kefirs are a great source of probiotics for people to consume in order to avoid Diverticular disease.

Prebiotics are another option when it comes to correcting the level of good/bad bacteria in the digestive system. These are substances that are known to develop and nurture the growth and development of the positive forms of bacteria that will keep you healthy and manage your wellbeing.

This is exactly what a person is looking for when they need to restore a healthy bacterial balance. One great probiotic is fructose-oligosaccharide powder but consult a doctor or doctor to learn about more prebiotics that can help in solving a poor bacterial balance and help to stop diverticulitis before it begins.

Stay away for foods high in fat. It is no secret that foods that are high in fat tend to slow down the digestion process and can lead to episodes of constipation. This is not healthy for the colon because it causes undue stress on the muscles and can cause long term damage to them. It is also much easier to maintain a healthy weight if the foods that are high in fat are avoided.

- Eat regularly

It is important to develop a normal eating schedule each day. It is believed that eating all of your snacks and meals at the same time each day will allow for your digestive system and colon to work in a more regular fashion and that will keep your colon in great shape and avoid the development of Diverticular disease. Make a goal to have your main three meals at about the same time each day along with any snacks. Most people are creatures of habit and this can become easy to do.

- Lean Meats

If you are going to consume meats, ensure that they are lean meats. Meats that have an excess of fatty tissue in them are not healthy for the digestion and they can introduce too much of the unhealthy kinds of bacteria in the colon, a perceived cause of diverticulitis. Some smart meats to eat are skinless poultry, pork loin and select lean cuts of steak.

- Gain an Understanding of Fiber and How It Affects Your Gut

Doctors that specialized in digestive tract illnesses have looked at what most people eat as a daily part of their diet and found that it is lacking in many of the essential nutrients that people should be eating for excellent digestive health. One of these ingredients is a diet that is much higher in fiber than is previously prescribed. One of the major contributors to the development of diverticulitis is that a person has difficulty in passing waste out of the colon through the rectum.

A diet high in fiber will make this much easier and alleviate much of the problem. After the muscles in a person's colon spend years straining to perform their function due to a diet that is low in fiber there is a development of this issue. Particularly in the United States this can be seen. Doctors start to realize that the colon is becoming a bit stretched which makes it even more difficult to pass excrement from the body and the stool needs to be even bulkier to be moved out without difficulty.

There was a study done by the Journal of Nutrition that observed nearly 45,000 health professionals participating in a long-term study. They learned that when a person ate a diet that was high in fiber, they lowered the risk of contracting Diverticular disease by somewhere in the neighborhood of 40%.

A high fiber diet presents a lot of other benefits as well. It fills your stomach easily and suppresses your appetite with can have a major assist in losing weight. Losing weight can help fight against developing Diverticular disease indirectly. Diverticular disease is much more likely to put a woman in the hospital if she is overweight or inactive. This is according to a study that was published in the American Journal of Gastroenterology.

It is recommended currently that 25 grams of fiber should be consumed by women each and every day. While men should eat even more fiber, being advised to try to consume about 38 grams of fiber in the daily diet. Even with these warnings the average American eats about 15 grams of fiber a woefully low portion. One of the best ways to augment your lack of fiber is to include foods that are high in fiber at every meal and also for snacks throughout the day.

Great sources of fiber for your diet include whole grains, oatmeal whole wheat bread, and barley. There are also some other great foods that you can dig into like lentils, fruits, vegetables and beans to give your diet a kick. One of the best snacking foods for a fiber input into your diet is to eat plenty of dried fruits which are a terrific source of fiber.

This type of eating plan is referred to as a whole foods diet because it includes a lot of foods that are not processed and treated with chemicals like white rice and white bread. Both of these are going to help cause diverticulitis rather than cure it. Eliminating the food that is bad for you is just as important as adding the food that is good for the body.

There are two types of fiber to consider soluble and insoluble. They are both an important part of a healthy diet but for different reasons. The insoluble fiber that is found in vegetable peels of fruit and seeds will add bulk to the stool in the colon and make it easier to pass reducing the wearing strain on the muscle. Soluble fiber is the other kind that a body needs, and it comes from foods like oatmeal, barley, and many fresh fruits like apples. This adds to the moisture located in the stool and that makes it easier to pass through the colon and reduces the strain.

The recommended intake of fiber is generally:

- Women age 19 to 50 = 25 grams per day
- Women age 50+ = 21 grams per day
- Men age 19 to 50 = 38 grams per day
- Men age 50+ = 30 grams per day

Please contact your doctor to confirm that these values are okay for your specific scenario.

- Drink More Fluids

Many overlook the importance of staying hydrated, but this tip may be the most effective in maintaining gut health. Drinking more fluids can help a high fiber diet be moved even easier through the digestive process with fewer chances of obstructions developing. Keeping the fluid intake into a normal level is all that is needed. There doesn't seem to be much of a benefit for drinking excessive liquids during the day. Look to drink as many non-calorie beverages as you can with your diet each day that means no limits to water or tea.

The recommended water intake is generally:

- Men age 19+ = 12 cups (about 3 liters) per day
- Women age 19+ = 9 cups (about 2 liters) per day

Please contact your doctor to confirm that these values are okay for your specific scenario.

Chapter 4. Clear Fluids Recipes

Breakfast

1. <u>Apple-Cinnamon Tea</u>

Preparation Time: 5 minutes

Cooking Time: 25 minutes

Servings: 4

Ingredients:

1 cup chopped apples, Honey Crisp, Fuji, Granny Smith, or Gala

3 cinnamon sticks

1 quart water

2 bags Earl Grey tea (caffeinated or decaffeinated)

1/3 cup honey, plus more if desired

Directions:

In a large saucepan over high heat, place the apples, cinnamon sticks, and water and bring to a boil. Lower the heat to medium and simmer for 15 minutes.

Remove from the heat and add the Earl Grey tea bags. Steep for 10 minutes.

Using a slotted spoon, remove the tea bags, apples, and cinnamon sticks. Add the honey and stir until it dissolves. Taste and add more honey, if desired. Serve hot.

Store leftovers in an airtight container in the refrigerator for up to 5 days. Enjoy cold or reheat in the microwave for 1 minute until hot.

Helpful Hint: Make this a ginger cinnamon tea by swapping the apples for ¼ cup minced fresh ginger and the Earl Grey tea for the zest and juice of 1 lemon (juice strained).

Nutrition: Calories: 101; Fat: <1g; Carbohydrates: 27g; Fiber: 1g; Protein: <1g; Sodium: 6mg; Vitamin B12: 0%; Iron: 1%

2. <u>Blueberry Green Tea</u>

Preparation Time: 5 minutes

Cooking Time: 15 minutes

Servings: 4

Ingredients:

½ cup fresh or frozen blueberries

1 quart water

2 bags green tea (caffeinated or decaffeinated)

1/3 cup honey, plus more if desired

Directions:

In a large saucepan over high heat, place the blueberries and water and bring to a boil. Lower the heat to medium and simmer for 5 minutes.

Remove from the heat and add the green tea bags. Steep for 10 minutes.

Using a slotted spoon, remove the tea bags and blueberries. Add the honey and stir until it dissolves. Taste and add more honey, if desired. Serve hot.

Store leftovers in an airtight container in the refrigerator for up to 5 days. Enjoy cold or reheat in the microwave for 1 minute until hot.

Nutrition: Calories: 95; Fat: 0g; Carbohydrates: 26g; Fiber: 1g; Protein: <1g; Sodium: 7mg; Vitamin B12: 0%; Iron: 1%

3. Citrus Sports Drink

Preparation Time: 5 minutes

Cooking Time: 0 minutes

Servings: 8

Ingredients:

4 cups coconut water

Juice of 4 large oranges (about 1½ cups), strained

2 tablespoons lemon juice, strained

2 tablespoons honey or maple syrup

1 teaspoon sea salt

Directions:

Place the coconut water, orange juice, lemon juice, honey, and salt in a jug or pitcher and stir until the salt is dissolved. Serve cold.

Store in the refrigerator for up to 5 days.

Nutrition: Calories: 59; Fat: <1g; Carbohydrates: 14g; Fiber: <1g; Protein: <1g; Sodium: 304mg; Vitamin B12: 0%; Iron: 1%

4. Homemade Orange Gelatin

Preparation Time: 10 minutes, plus 4 hours chilling time

Cooking Time: 3 minutes

Servings: 4

Ingredients:

Juice of 8 large oranges (about 3 cups), strained and divided

2 tablespoons unflavored gelatin

2 tablespoons honey or maple syrup

Directions:

In a large bowl, pour in ½ cup of orange juice and sprinkle with gelatin. Whisk well and let sit for 5 minutes, until the gelatin begins to set but is not quite smooth.

In a medium saucepan over low heat, pour in the remaining 2½ cups of orange juice and cook until just before boiling, 2 to 3 minutes.

Remove from the heat and pour the hot juice into the gelatin mixture. Add the honey or maple syrup and stir until the gelatin is dissolved.

Pour into an 8-by-8-inch baking dish and transfer to the refrigerator. Refrigerate for 4 hours to set. Serve cold.

To store, cover the dish with plastic wrap and refrigerate for up to 5 days.

Helpful Hint: Swap the fruit juice in this gelatin for a number of different flavors. I recommend lemon, lime, or even peach. Just be sure your fruit juice is pulp-free.

Nutrition: Calories: 127; Fat: <1g; Carbohydrates: 28g; Fiber: <1g; Protein: 6g; Sodium: 2mg; Vitamin B12: 0%; Iron: 2%

5. Raspberry Lemonade Ice Pops

Preparation Time: 10 minutes, plus 4 hours chilling time

Cooking Time: 0 minutes

Servings: Makes 4 ice pops

Ingredients:

3 cups frozen raspberries

1 teaspoon lemon juice, strained

¼ cup coconut water

¼ cup honey or maple syrup

Directions:

In a blender, puree the raspberries, lemon juice, and coconut water until smooth.

Pour the mixture through a fine mesh strainer into a bowl to remove the seeds. Stir in the honey until well mixed.

Divide the mixture equally among 4 popsicle molds and freeze until solid, 3 to 4 hours.

Helpful Hint: You may want to stock up on ice pop molds during warmer months, as they can be hard to find in the winter.

Nutrition: Calories: 120; Fat: 0g; Carbohydrates: 31g; Fiber: 7g; Protein: 2g; Sodium: 2mg; Vitamin B12: 0%; Iron: 1%

6. Homemade No Pulp Orange Juice

Preparation Time: 5 mins.

Cooking Time: 0 mins.

Servings: 1 ½ cups

Ingredients:

Oranges (4)

Directions:

Lightly squeeze the oranges on a hard surface to soften the exterior. Slice each in half.

Squeeze each orange over a fine mesh strainer.

Gently press the pulp to extract all possible liquid.

Serve over ice. Enjoy!

Nutrition:

50 calories, 0.2 g fat, 11.5 g carbs, g fiber, 0.8 g protein

7. Apple Orange Juice

Preparation Time: 5 mins.

Cooking Time: 0 mins.

Servings: 2

Ingredients:

Apple (1 Gala, peeled, cored, sliced)

Oranges (2, peeled, halved, seeded)

Honey (2 tsp, optional)

Water (3/4 cup)

Directions:

Squeeze each orange over a fine mesh strainer.

Gently press the pulp to extract as much liquid as possible.

Add in your apple, water, and orange juice in your blender and blend.

Set a fine mesh strainer a bowl. Before transferring your juice into the strainer.

Once again, gently press the pulp to remove all possible liquid then discard pulp.

Stir in your honey then serve over ice.

Nutrition:

180 calories, 1 g fat, 43 g carbs, 1 g fiber, 2 g protein

8. Pineapple Mint Juice

Preparation Time: 5 mins.

Cooking Time: 0 mins.

Servings: 4

Ingredients:

pineapple (3 cups, cored and sliced, chunks)

mint leaves (10 to 12, or to taste)

sugar, or to taste (2 tablespoons, optional)

water (1 1/2 cups)

ice cubes (1 cup)

Directions:

Add all your ingredients into your blender, and blend.

Set a fine mesh strainer a bowl. Before transferring your juice into the strainer.

Gently press the pulp to extract all possible liquid then discard pulp.

Serve over ice. Enjoy!

Nutrition:

78 calories, 1 g fat, 22 g carbs, 2 g fiber, 1 g protein

9. Celery Apple Juice

Preparation Time: 5 mins.

Cooking Time: 0 mins.

Servings: 2

Ingredients:

Celery (12 stalks, peeled, chopped)

Apple (peeled, cored, seeded, sliced)

Ginger (1-inch root, peeled, chopped)

Lemon (1/4, juiced)

Water (2 cups)

Directions:

Add all your ingredients into your blender, and blend.

Set a fine mesh strainer a bowl. Before transferring your juice into the strainer.

Gently press the pulp to extract all possible liquid then discard pulp.

Serve over ice. Enjoy!

Nutrition:

119 calories, 1 g fat, 29 g carbs, 7 g fiber, 2 g protein

10.   Homemade Banana Apple Juice

Preparation Time: 10 mins.

Cooking Time: 0 mins.

Servings: 2

Ingredients:

Bananas (2, peeled, sliced)

Apple (1/2, peeled, cored and chopped)

Honey (1 tbsp.)

Water (1½ cups)

Directions:

Add all your ingredients into your blender, and blend.

Set a fine mesh strainer a bowl. Before transferring your juice into the strainer.

Gently press the pulp to extract all possible liquid then discard pulp.

Serve over ice. Enjoy!

Nutrition:

132 calories, 2 g fat, 27 g carbs, 3 g fiber, 4 g protein

11.   Sweet Detox Juice

Preparation Time: 10 mins.

Cooking Time: 0 mins.

Servings: 2

Ingredients:

baby spinach (2 cups, chopped)

parsley (1 handful, chopped)

apple (1, green, peeled, cored, seeded, sliced0

cucumber (1 large English, seeded, chopped)

ginger (1-inch, peeled)

lemon (1, juiced)

Directions:

Add all your ingredients into your blender, and blend.

Set a fine mesh strainer a bowl. Before transferring your juice into the strainer.

Gently press the pulp to extract all possible liquid then discard pulp.

Serve over ice. Enjoy!

Nutrition:

209 calories, 2 g fat, 48 g carbs, 17 g fiber, 12 g protein

12.   Pineapple Ginger Juice

Preparation Time: 35 mins.

Cooking Time: 0 mins.

Servings: 7 cups

Ingredients:

pineapple (10 cups, chopped)

water (6 cups)

Apples (3, Fuji, chopped)

ginger (4-inch root, peeled, chopped)

lemon juice (1/4 cup)

sugar (1/4 cup)

Directions:

Add all your ingredients into your blender, and blend.

Set a fine mesh strainer a bowl. Before transferring your juice into the strainer.

Gently press the pulp to extract all possible liquid then discard pulp.

Serve over ice. Enjoy!

Nutrition:

71 calories, 1 g fat, 20 g carbs, 3 g fiber, 1 g protein

13. Carrot Orange Juice

Preparation Time: 15 mins.

Cooking Time: 0 mins.

Servings: 2

Ingredients:

Tomato (1, yellow, medium), cut into wedges

Orange (1, peeled, quartered)

Apple (1, peeled, cored, chopped)

Carrots (4, jumbo, peeled, chopped)

Water (2 cups)

Directions:

Add all your ingredients into your blender, and blend.

Set a fine mesh strainer a bowl. Before transferring your juice into the strainer.

Gently press the pulp to extract all possible liquid then discard pulp.

Serve over ice. Enjoy!

Nutrition:

111 calories, 1 g fat, 24 g carbs, 1 g fiber, 2 g protein

14. Strawberry Apple Juice

Preparation Time: 5 mins.

Cooking Time: 0 mins.

Servings: 8-10 oz

Ingredients:

Strawberries (2 cups, tops removed)

Apple (1, red, peeled, seeded, cored, chopped)

chia seeds (1 tbsp.)

Water (1 cup)

Directions:

Add all your ingredients into your blender, and blend.

Set a fine mesh strainer a bowl. Before transferring your juice into the strainer.

Gently press the pulp to extract all possible liquid then discard pulp.

Add in your chia seeds then leave to sit for at least 5 minutes.

Serve over ice. Enjoy!

Nutrition:

245 calories, 5 g fat, 52 g carbs, 7 g fiber, 4 g protein

15. Autumn Energizer Juice

Preparation Time: 10 mins.

Cooking Time: 0 mins.

Servings: 2

Ingredients:

Pears (2, peeled, seeded, chopped)

Apples (2, Ambrosia, peeled, cored, chopped)

Apples (2, Granny Smith, peeled, cored, chopped)

Mandarins (2, juiced)

sweet potato (2 cups, peeled, chopped)

cape gooseberries (1 pint)

ginger (2-inch root, peeled)

Directions:

Add all your ingredients into your blender, and blend.

Set a fine mesh strainer a bowl. Before transferring your juice into the strainer.

Gently press the pulp to extract all possible liquid then discard pulp.

Serve over ice. Enjoy!

Nutrition:

170 calories, 3 g fat, 33 g carbs, 9 g fiber, 4 g protein

Lunch

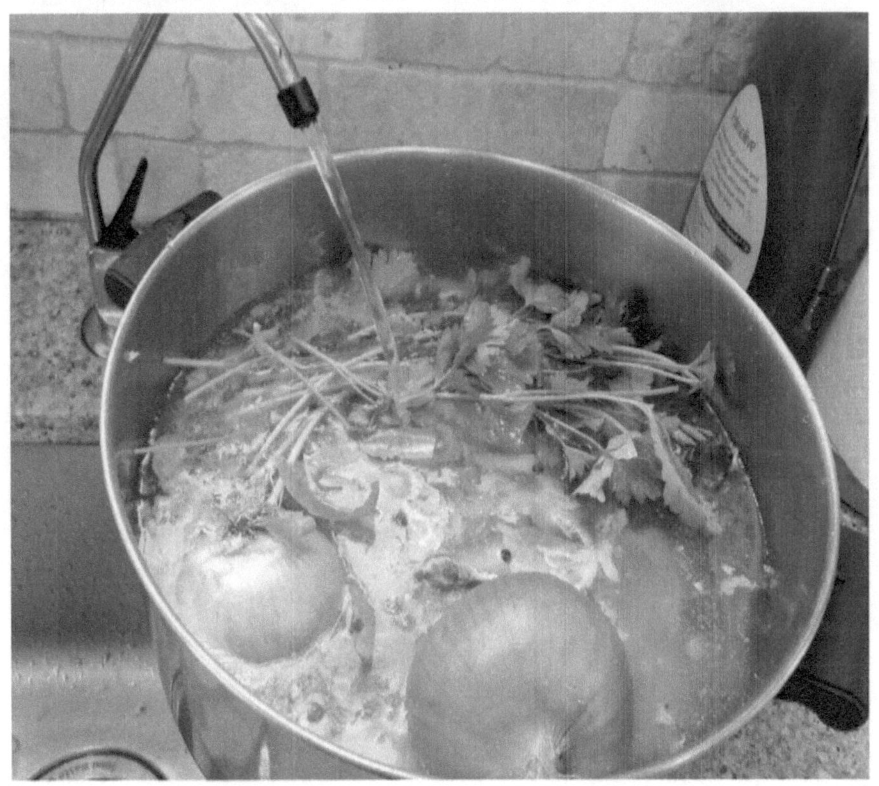

16.   Slow Cooker Pork Bone Broth

Preparation Time: 15 mins.

Cooking Time: 24 hours + roasting time

Servings: 12 cups

Ingredients:

pork bones (2 pounds – roasted)

onion (½ chopped)

carrots (2 medium chopped)

celery (1 stalk chopped)

garlic whole (2 cloves)

bay leaf (1)

sea salt (1 tablespoon)

peppercorns (1 teaspoon)

Apple Cider Vinegar (¼ cup)

Filtered water

Directions

Transfer your ingredients to your slow cooker. Top with enough water to cover then allow to slowly come to a boil on high heat.

Switch to low heat and simmer for at least 24 hours on low. (The longer it cooks, the more flavor you will get.)

Carefully pour the mixture through a fine mesh strainer into a large bowl. Taste and season with salt.

Serve hot. Enjoy!

Nutrition:

65 calories, 2 g fat, 7 g carbs, 4 g fiber, 6 g protein

17.   Homemade Chicken Stock

Preparation Time: 10 minutes

Cooking Time: 2½ to 12½ hours

Servings: 6

Ingredients:

1 (2-pound) chicken carcass

5 celery stalks, chopped

4 carrots, chopped

1 white or Spanish onion, chopped

2 garlic cloves, crushed

2 bay leaves

1 teaspoon dried thyme

1 teaspoon dried sage

1 teaspoon black peppercorns

Salt

Directions:

Preheat the oven to 425°F.

On a large baking sheet, spread out the chicken bones, celery, carrots, onion, garlic, and bay leaves. Sprinkle the thyme, sage, and peppercorns over the top. Roast for 20 to 30 minutes, or until the vegetables and bones have a rich brown color.

Transfer the roasted bones and vegetables to a large stockpot. Add 6 quarts of water and slowly bring to a boil over high heat. Lower the heat to medium-low and simmer for at least 2 hours and up to 12 hours. (The longer it cooks, the more flavor you will get.)

Carefully pour the mixture through a fine mesh strainer into a large bowl. Season with salt and serve hot.

Store in airtight containers in the refrigerator for up to 5 days or in the freezer for up to 4 months.

Helpful Hint: Feel free to combine all the ingredients in a slow cooker instead. Before you go to bed, set it on high, and strain the stock the next morning.

Nutrition: Calories: 33; Fat: 1g; Carbohydrates: 3g; Fiber: 0g; Protein: 3g; Sodium: 20mg; Vitamin B12: 0%; Iron: 0%

18.   Best Homemade Broth

Cooking Time: 2 hours 5 minutes

Preparation Time: 15 minutes

Servings: 8

Ingredients:

1 (3-lb.) chicken, cut into pieces

5 medium carrots, peeled and cut into 2-inch pieces

4 celery stalks with leaves, cut into 2-inch pieces

6 fresh thyme sprigs

6 fresh parsley sprigs

Salt, to taste

9 C. cold water

Directions:

In a large pan, add all the ingredients over medium-high heat and bring to a boil.

Reduce the heat to medium-low and simmer, covered for about 2 hours, skimming the foam from the surface occasionally.

Through a fine-mesh sieve, strain the broth into a large bowl.

Serve hot.

Nutrition:

Calories per serving: 275; Carbohydrates: 4.3g; Protein: 49.7g; Fat: 5.2g; Sugar: 2g; Sodium: 160mg; Fiber: 1.2g

19.   Clean Testing Broth

Cooking Time: 15 minutes

Preparation Time: 5 hours 50 minutes

Servings: 10

Ingredients:

4 lb. chicken bones

Salt, to taste

10 C. filtered water

2 tbsp. apple cider vinegar

1 lemon, quartered

3 bay leaves

3 tsp. ground turmeric

2 tbsp. peppercorns

Directions:

Preheat the oven to 400 degrees F.

Arrange the bones onto a large baking sheet and sprinkle with salt.

Roast for about 45 minutes.

Remove from the oven and transfer the bones into a large pan.

Add the remaining ingredients and stir to combine.

Place the pan over medium-high heat and bring to a boil.

Reduce the heat to low and simmer, covered for about 4-5 hours, skimming the foam from the surface occasionally.

Through a fine-mesh sieve, strain the broth into a large bowl.

Serve hot.

Nutrition:

Calories per serving: 140; Carbohydrates: 0.6g; Protein: 25g; Fat: 2.6g; Sugar: 0.1g; Sodium: 73mg; Fiber: 0.1g

20.   Healing Broth

Cooking Time: 15 minutes

Preparation Time: 10 hours 25 minutes

Servings: 12

Ingredients:

3 tbsp. extra-virgin olive oil

2½ lb. chicken bones

4 celery stalks, chopped roughly

3 large carrots, peeled and chopped roughly

1 bay leaf

1 tbsp. black peppercorns

2 whole cloves

1 tbsp. apple cider vinegar

Warm water, as required

Directions:

In a Dutch oven, heat the oil over medium-high heat and sear the bones or about 3-5 minutes or until browned.

With a slotted spoon, transfer the bones into a bowl.

In the same pan, add the celery stalks and carrots and cook for about 15 minutes, stirring occasionally.

Add browned bones, bay leaf, black peppercorns, cloves and vinegar and stir to combine.

Add the enough warm water to cover the bones mixture completely and bring to a gentle boil.

Reduce the heat to low and simmer, covered for about 8-10 hours, skimming the foam from the surface occasionally.

Through a fine-mesh sieve, strain the broth into a large bowl.

Serve hot.

Nutrition:

Calories per serving: 67; Carbohydrates: 2g; Protein: 5.7g; Fat: 4.1g; Sugar: 1g; Sodium: 29mg; Fiber: 0.5g

21. Veggie Lover's Broth

Cooking Time: 15 minutes

Preparation Time: 2 hours 5 minutes

Servings: 10

Ingredients:

4 carrots, peeled and chopped roughly

4 celery stalks, chopped roughly

3 parsnips, peeled and chopped roughly

2 large potatoes, peeled and chopped roughly

1 medium beet, trimmed and chopped roughly

1 large bunch fresh parsley

1 (1-inch) piece fresh ginger, sliced

Filtered water, as required

Directions:

In a large pan, add all the ingredients over medium-high heat.

Add enough water to cover the veggie mixture and bring to a boil.

Reduce the heat to low and simmer, covered for about 2-3 hours.

Through a fine-mesh sieve, strain the broth into a large bowl.

Serve hot.

Nutrition:

Calories per serving: 82; Carbohydrates: 19g; Protein: 1.9g; Fat: 0.2g; Sugar: 3.9g; Sodium: 37mg; Fiber: 3.7g

22. Brain Healthy Broth

Cooking Time: 10 minutes

Preparation Time: 12 hours 5 minutes

Servings: 6

Ingredients:

12 C. filtered water

2 lb. non-oily fish heads and bones

¼ C. apple cider vinegar

Sea salt, to taste

Directions:

In a large pan, add all the ingredients over medium-high heat.

Add enough water to cover the veggie mixture and bring to a boil.

Reduce the heat to low and simmer, covered for about 10-12 hours, skimming the foam from the surface occasionally.

Through a fine-mesh sieve, strain the broth into a large bowl.

Serve hot.

Nutrition:

Calories per serving: 75; Carbohydrates: 0.1g; Protein: 13.4g; Fat: 1.7g; Sugar: 0g; Sodium: 253mg; Fiber: 0g

23.   Minerals Rich Broth

Cooking Time: 2 hours 25 minutes

Preparation Time: 15 minutes

Servings: 8

Ingredients:

5-7 lb. non-oily fish carcasses and heads

2 tbsp. olive oil

3 carrots, scrubbed and chopped roughly

2 celery stalks, chopped roughly

1 bay leaf

2 whole cloves

2 tsp. peppercorns

1 bunch fresh parsley

4 fresh thyme stems

Directions:

In a large pan, heat the oil over medium-low heat and cook the carrots and celery for about 20 minutes, stirring occasionally.

Add the fish bones and enough water to cover by 1-inch and stir to combine.

Increase the heat to medium-high and bring to a boil.

Reduce the heat to low and simmer, covered for about 1-2 hours, skimming the foam from the surface occasionally.

Through a fine-mesh sieve, strain the broth into a large bowl.

Serve hot.

Nutrition:

Calories per serving: 113; Carbohydrates: 2.5g; Protein: 13.7g; Fat: 5.2g; Sugar: 1.2g; Sodium: 234mg; Fiber: 0.7g

24.   Holiday Favorite Gelatin

Preparation Time: 15 minutes

Cooking Time: 0 minutes

Servings: 6

Ingredients:

1 tbsp. grass-fed gelatin powder

1¾ C. fresh apple juice, warmed

¼ C. boiling water

1-2 drops fresh lemon juice

Directions:

In a medium bowl, pour in the tbsp. of gelatin powder.

Add just enough warm apple juice to cover the gelatin and stir well.

Set aside for about 2-3 minutes or until it forms a thick syrup.

Add ¼ C. of the boiling water and stir until gelatin is dissolved completely.

Add the remaining juice and lemon juice and stir well.

Transfer the mixture into a parchment paper-lined baking dish and refrigerate for 2 hours or until the top is firm before serving.

Nutrition:

Calories per serving: 40; Carbohydrates: 8.2g; Protein: 1.9g; Fat: 0.1g; Sugar: 7g; Sodium: 5mg; Fiber: 0.2g

25.   Homemade Beef Stock

Preparation Time: 10 minutes

Cooking Time: 2½ to 12½ hours

Servings: 6

Ingedients:

2 pounds beef bones (preferably with marrow)

5 celery stalks, chopped

4 carrots, chopped

1 white or Spanish onion, chopped

2 garlic cloves, crushed

2 bay leaves

1 teaspoon dried thyme

1 teaspoon dried sage

1 teaspoon black peppercorns

Salt

Directions:

Preheat the oven to 425°F.

On a large baking sheet, spread out the beef bones, celery, carrots, onion, garlic, and bay leaves. Sprinkle the thyme, sage, and peppercorns over the top.

Roast for 20 to 30 minutes, or until the vegetables and bones have a rich brown color.

Transfer the roasted bones and vegetables to a large stockpot. Cover with water and slowly bring to a boil over high heat. Lower the heat to medium-low and simmer for at least 2 hours and up to 12 hours. (The longer it cooks, the more flavor you will get.)

Carefully pour the mixture through a fine mesh strainer into a large bowl. Taste and season with salt. Serve hot.

Store in airtight containers in the refrigerator for up to 5 days or in the freezer for up to 4 months.

Helpful Hint: You can also make this stock in a slow cooker set on high. I typically start cooking my stock in the late evening, and I strain it when I wake up the next morning.

Nutrition: Calories: 37; Fat: 1g; Carbohydrates: 3g; Fiber: 0g; Protein: 4g;

Sodium: 58mg; Vitamin B12: 0%; Iron: 0%

Snack

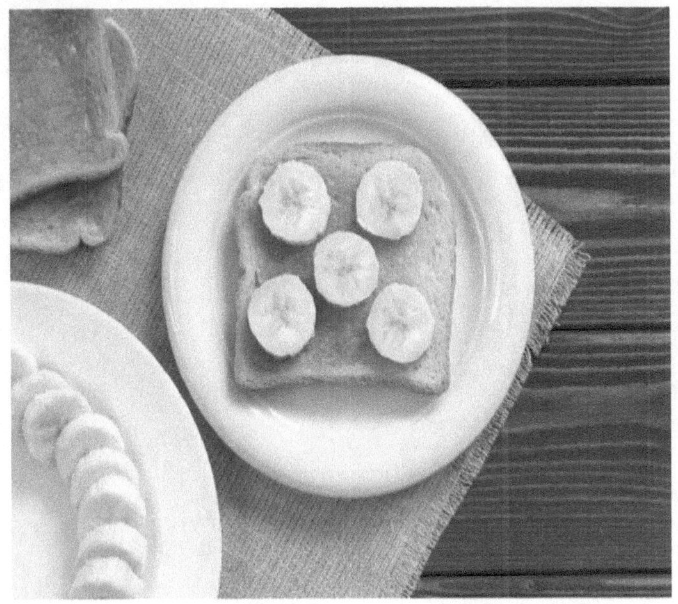

26.   3-Ingredient Sugar Free Gelatin

Preparation Time: 5 mins.

Cooking Time: 4hrs.

Servings:6-8

Ingredients:

Water (1/4 cup, room temperature)

Water (1/4 cup, hot)

Gelatin (1 tbsp.)

Orange Juice (1 cup, unsweetened)

Directions:

Combine your gelatin and room temperature water, stirring until fully dissolved.

Stir in your hot water then leave to rest for about 2 minutes.

Add in your juice and stir until combined.

Transfer to serving size containers then place on a tray in the refrigerator to set for about 4 hours.

Enjoy!

Nutrition:

17 calories, 0 g fat, 4 g carbs, 0 g fiber, 0 g protein

27.   Cran - Kombucha Jell-O

Preparation Time: 5 mins.

Cooking Time: 4hrs.

Servings: 6

Ingredients:

Water (1/4 cup, room temperature)

Hot Water (1/4 cup)

Gelatin (1 tbsp.)

Cranberry kombucha (1 cup, unsweetened)

Directions:

Combine your gelatin and room temperature water, stirring until fully dissolved.

Stir in your hot water then leave to rest for about 2 minutes.

Add in your kombucha and stir until combined.

Transfer to serving size containers then place on a tray in the refrigerator to set for about 4 hours.

Enjoy!

Nutrition:

13 calories, 0 g fat, 1 g carbs, 0 g fiber, 0 g protein

28.   Strawberry Gummies

Preparation Time: 5 mins.

Cooking Time: 4 hrs.

Servings: 20-40 mini gummies

Ingredients:

Strawberries (1 cup, hulled, chopped)

Water (3/4 cup)

Gelatin (2 tbsp.)

Directions:

Set your water and berries on to boil on high heat. /remove from heat as soon as the mixture begins to boil.

Transfer to your blender and blend. Add in your gelatin then blend once more.

Pour your mixture into a silicone gummy mold.

Place on a tray in the refrigerator to set for about 4 hours.

Enjoy!

Nutrition:

3 calories, 0 g fat, 0 g carbs, 0 g fiber, 0 g protein

29.   Fruity Jell-O Stars

Preparation Time: 15 mins.

Cooking Time: 5 mins.

Servings: 4

Ingredients:

Gelatin (1 Tbsp, powdered)

Boiling Water (3/4 cup)

Fruit (3 ½ cups)

Honey (1 Tbsp)

Lemon Juice (1 Tsp.)

Directions:

Add all your ingredients into your blender and blend. Add in your gelatin then blend once more.

Pour your mixture into a silicone gummy mold.

Place on a tray in the refrigerator to set for about 4 hours.

Enjoy!

Nutrition:

73 calories, 2 g fat, 14 g carbs, 0 g fiber, 1 g protein

30. Plum and Nectarine Gelatin Pudding

Preparation Time: 15 mins.

Cooking Time: 0 mins.

Servings: 5

Ingredients:

Nectarine (1, large)

Plums (2, small)

Gelatin (2 tbsp.)

Water (1 1/2 cup, room temp.)

Boiling water (2 cups)

lemon juice (2 tsp.)

Honey (1/3 cup)

Vanilla (1 tsp.)

sea salt (1/8 tsp.)

Directions:

Add your fruits in your blend to puree until smooth with room temperature water, lemon juice and vanilla until smooth.

Strain through a fine mesh strainer.

Combine your gelatin and fruit mixture, stirring until fully dissolved.

Stir in your hot water then leave to rest for about 2 minutes.

Add in your remaining ingredients and stir until combined.

Transfer to serving size containers then place on a tray in the refrigerator to set for about 4 hours.

Enjoy!

Nutrition:

157 calories, 5g fat, 26 g carbs, 1 g fiber, 3 g protein

31.   Homemade Lemon Gelatin

Preparation Time: 2 hrs. 5 mins.

Cooking Time: 0 mins.

Servings: 8

Ingredients:

Gelatin (3 tbsp., granulated)

Stevia (1½ cup)

Boiling Water (1 1/2 cups)

Cold Water (3 cups)

Lemon Juice (1 1/8 cups)

Lemon zest (1/2 tsp)

Directions:

Combine your gelatin and room temperature water, stirring until fully dissolved.

Stir in your hot water then leave to rest for about 2 minutes.

Add in your remaining ingredients and stir until combined.

Transfer to serving size containers then place on a tray in the refrigerator to set for about 4 hours.

Enjoy!

Nutrition:

68 calories, 0 g fat, 1 g carbs, 0 g fiber, 2 g protein

32.   Sour Blueberry Gummies

Preparation Time: 5 mins.

Cooking Time: 5 mins.

Servings: 9

Ingredients:

Blueberries (1 1/2 cup)

lemon juice (1 cup)

honey (3 tbsp)

gelatin (1/3 cup, grass-fed)

Directions:

Set your water and berries on to boil on high heat. /remove from heat as soon as the mixture begins to boil.

Transfer to your blender and blend. Add in your gelatin then blend once more.

Pour your mixture into a silicone gummy mold.

Place on a tray in the refrigerator to set for about 4 hours.

Enjoy!

Nutrition:

73 calories, 2 g fat, 14 g carbs, 0 g fiber, 1 g protein

33.   Sugar – Free Cinnamon Jelly

Preparation Time: 2 hrs. 15 mins.

Cooking Time: 0 mins.

Servings: 2

Ingredients:

Hot Herbal Tea (1 cup)

Room Temperature Water (1 cup)

Gelatin (2 tsp)

Sweetener(1/3 cup)

Directions:

Combine your gelatin and room temperature water, stirring until fully dissolved.

Stir in your hot water then leave to rest for about 2 minutes.

Add in your juice and stir until combined.

Transfer to serving size containers then place on a tray in the refrigerator to set for about 4 hours.

Enjoy!

Nutrition:

35 calories, 0 g fat, 17 g carbs, 0 g fiber, 0 g protein

Dinner

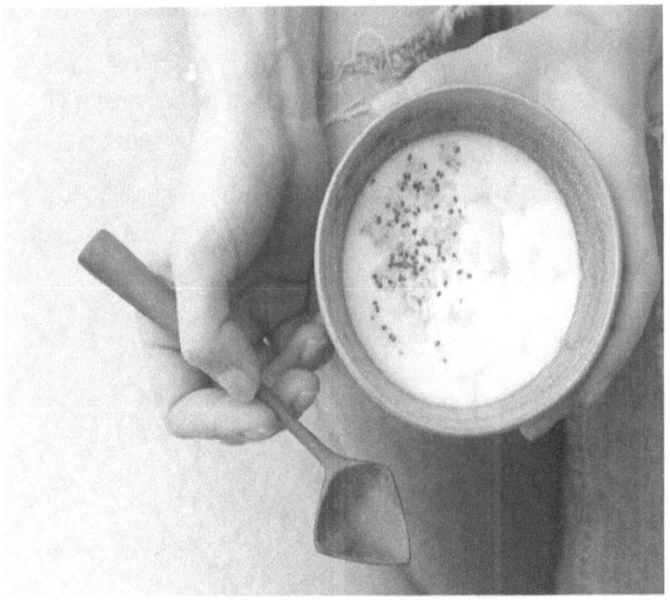

34.   Homey Clear Chicken Broth

Preparation Time: 10 mins.

Cooking Time: 3-1/4 hours

Servings: 6 cups

Ingredients:

Chicken neck (2 lbs)

celery ribs with leaves (2, cut into chunks)

carrots (2 medium, cut into chunks)

onions (2 medium, quartered)

bay leaves (2)

rosemary (1/2 teaspoon dried, crushed)

thyme (1/2 teaspoon dried)

peppercorns (8 to 10 whole)

cold water (2 quarts)

Directions:

Transfer the bones and vegetables to your stockpot. Top with enough water to cover then allow to slowly come to a boil on high heat.

Switch to low heat and simmer for at least 2 hours and up to 12 hours. (The longer it cooks, the more flavor you will get.)

Carefully pour the mixture through a fine mesh strainer into a large bowl. Taste and season with salt.

Serve hot.

Nutrition:

245 calories, 14g fat, 8g carbs, 2g fiber, 21g protein

35. Asian Inspired Wonton Broth

Preparation Time: 5 mins.

Cooking Time: 1 hour 35 mins.

Servings: 1-gallon

Ingredients:

chicken thigh (1, skin on)

carrot (1, coarsely chopped)

celery (1 stalk, coarsely chopped)

onion (1 small, quartered)

ginger (3 dime-sized pieces)

Kosher salt (2 tablespoons)

Turmeric (1/4 teaspoon)

MSG, (1/8 teaspoon, don't leave it out)

Peppercorns (5 white, black can be substituted)

Water (1 gallon)

Directions:

Transfer all your ingredients to your stockpot. Top with enough water to cover then allow to slowly come to a boil on high heat.

Switch to low heat and simmer for at least 1 hours and 30 minutes.

Carefully pour the mixture through a fine mesh strainer into a large bowl. Taste and season with salt.

Serve hot.

Nutrition:

181 calories, 7 g fat, 14 g carbs, 1 g fiber, 14g protein

36.   Mushroom, Cauliflower & Cabbage Broth

Preparation Time: 10 mins.

Cooking Time: 50 mins.

Servings: 3

Ingredients:

yellow onion (1 large)

celery stalks (1 cup, chopped)

carrots (2 diced or cubed)

French beans (10)

cabbage (½ diced)

celery leaves (1 to 2 stalks)

mushrooms sliced (1½ cup)

cauliflower (8 florets)

garlic (1 tsp, chopped)

ginger (1 tsp, chopped)

oil (1 tbsp)

scallions (1 stalk)

pepper (½ tsp crushed)

Directions:

Transfer all your ingredients to your stockpot. Top with enough water to cover then allow to slowly come to a boil on high heat.

Switch to low heat and simmer for 50 minutes.

Carefully pour the mixture through a fine mesh strainer into a large bowl. Mash the veggies well to extract all their juices.

Taste and season with salt. Enjoy.

Nutrition:

141 calories, 5g fat, 22g carbs, 7 g fiber, 5 g protein

37.   Oxtail Bone Broth

Preparation Time: 15 mins.

Cooking Time: 12 hours

Servings: 8 cups

Ingredients:

Oxtail (2 Pounds)

Onion (1, chopped in quarters)

celery stalks (2, chopped in half)

carrots (2, chopped in half)

garlic cloves (3, whole)

bay leaves (2)

apple cider vinegar (2 Tablespoons)

salt (1 Tablespoon)

peppercorns (1/2 Tablespoon)

filtered water (enough to cover bones)

Directions:

Transfer the bones and vegetables to your stockpot. Top with enough water to cover then allow to slowly come to a boil on high heat.

Switch to low heat and simmer for at least 2 hours and up to 12 hours. (The longer it cooks, the more flavor you will get.)

Carefully pour the mixture through a fine mesh strainer into a large bowl. Taste and season with salt.

Serve hot.

Nutrition:

576 calories, 48 g fat, 8 g carbs, 0 g fiber, 24 g protein

38. Beef Bone Broth

Preparation Time: 15 mins.

Cooking Time: 12 hours

Servings: 8 cups

Ingredients:

beef bones (2 Pounds)

onion (1, chopped in quarters)

celery stalks (2, chopped in half)

carrots (2, chopped in half)

garlic cloves (3, whole)

bay leaves (2)

apple cider vinegar (2 Tablespoons)

salt (1 Tablespoon)

peppercorns (1/2 Tablespoon)

filtered water (enough to cover bones)

Directions:

Transfer the bones and vegetables to your stockpot. Top with enough water to cover then allow to slowly come to a boil on high heat.

Switch to low heat and simmer for at least 2 hours and up to 12 hours. (The longer it cooks, the more flavor you will get.)

Carefully pour the mixture through a fine mesh strainer into a large bowl. Taste and season with salt.

Serve hot.

Nutrition:

69 calories, 4 g fat, 1 g carbs, 0.1 g fiber, 6 g protein

39. Ginger, Mushroom & Cauliflower Broth

Preparation Time: 10 mins.

Cooking Time: 50 mins.

Servings: 3

Ingredients:

1 large yellow onion

1 cup celery stalks chopped

2 carrots diced or cubed

10 French beans

1 ginger root, peeled and diced or grated

1 to 2 stalks celery leaves or coriander leaves

1½ cup mushrooms sliced

8 florets cauliflower

1 tsp garlic chopped

1 tbsp oil

1 stalk spring onion greens or scallions

½ tsp crushed pepper or ground pepper

Directions:

Transfer your ingredients to your stockpot. Top with enough water to cover then allow to slowly come to a boil on high heat.

Switch to low heat and simmer for at least 50 minutes on low hat.

Carefully pour the mixture through a fine mesh strainer into a large bowl. Taste and season with salt.

Serve hot. Enjoy!

Nutrition:

141 calories, 5 g fat, 22 g carbs, 7 g fiber, 5 g protein

40. Pork Stock

Preparation Time: 15 mins.

Cooking Time: 12 hours

Servings: 8 cups

Ingredients:

pork bones (2 Pounds, roasted)

onion (1, chopped in quarters)

celery stalks (2, chopped in half)

carrots (2, chopped in half)

garlic cloves (3, whole)

bay leaves (2)

apple cider vinegar (2 Tablespoons)

salt (1 Tablespoon)

peppercorns (1/2 Tablespoon)

filtered water (enough to cover bones)

Directions:

Transfer the bones and vegetables to your stockpot. Top with enough water to cover then allow to slowly come to a boil on high heat.

Switch to low heat and simmer for 12 hours on low. (The longer it cooks, the more flavor you will get.)

Carefully pour the mixture through a fine mesh strainer into a large bowl. Taste and season with salt.

Serve hot. Enjoy!

Nutrition:

69 calories, 4 g fat, 1 g carbs, 0.1 g fiber, 6 g protein

41.   Fish Broth

Preparation Time: 15 mins.

Cooking Time: 45 mins.

Servings: 32

Ingredients:

olive oil (3 tablespoons)

onion (1 large, chopped)

carrot (1 large, chopped)

fennel bulb (1, chopped, optional)

celery stalks (3, chopped)

Salt

white wine (2 cups)

fish bones and heads (2 to 5 pounds)

mushrooms (A handful of dried, optional)

bay leaves (2 to 4)

1-star anise pod (optional)

Thyme (1 to 2 teaspoons dried or fresh)

kombu kelp (3 or 4 pieces of dried, optional)

Chopped fronds from the fennel bulb

Directions:

Transfer the bones and vegetables to your stockpot. Top with enough water to cover then allow to slowly come to a boil on high heat.

Switch to low heat and simmer for 45 mins.

Carefully pour the mixture through a fine mesh strainer into a large bowl. Taste and season with salt.

Serve hot. Enjoy!

Nutrition:

29 calories, 1 g fat, 2 g carbs, 1 g fiber, 1 g protein

42.   Indian Inspired Vegetable stock

Preparation Time: 15 mins.

Cooking Time: 11 mins.

Servings: 3 cups

Ingredients:

Onions (3/4 cup, roughly chopped)

Carrot (3/4 cup, roughly chopped)

Tomatoes (3/4 cup, roughly chopped)

Potatoes (3/4 cup, roughly chopped)

Turmeric (1 tsp.)

salt to taste

Directions:

Transfer your ingredients to your stockpot. Top with enough water to cover then allow to slowly come to a boil on high heat.

Switch to low heat and simmer for 11 minutes.

Carefully pour the mixture through a fine mesh strainer into a large bowl.

Taste and season with salt.

Serve hot. Enjoy!

Nutrition:

103 calories, 0.2mg fat, 23.3 g carbs, 3.1 g fiber, 2.2 g protein

43. Clear Pumpkin Broth

Preparation Time: 15 mins.

Cooking Time: 30 mins.

Servings: 6 cups

Ingredients:

instant dashi powder (3 teaspoons)

sake or dry sherry (1 cup)

mirin (2 tablespoons)

soy sauce (1 cup)

sugar (2 tablespoons)

water (6 cups)

ginger (2 tablespoons, minced)

potatoes (2 cups, peeled and diced)

kabocha (3 cups, peeled and diced)

carrot (1, peeled and diced)

onion (1, diced)

scallions (½ cup, chopped)

Directions:

Transfer the bones and vegetables to your stockpot. Top with enough water to cover then allow to slowly come to a boil on high heat.

Switch to low heat and simmer for at least 30 minutes

Carefully pour the mixture through a fine mesh strainer into a large bowl. Taste and season with salt.

Serve hot. Enjoy!

Nutrition:

216 calories, 1 g fat, 37 g carbs, 4 g fiber, 8 g protein

Dessert

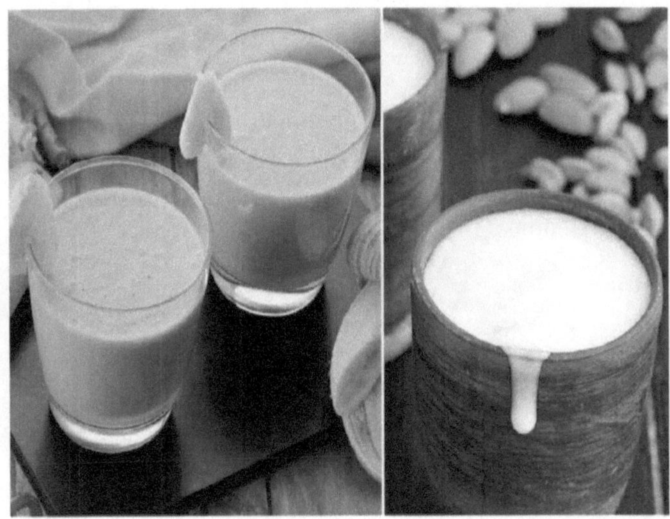

44. Tropical Fruit Punch

Preparation Time: 3 mins.

Cooking Time: 0 mins.

Servings: 4 glasses

Ingredients:

Pineapple (1, peeled, cored, sliced)

Apples (2, peeled, cored, quartered)

Oranges (2, juiced)

Pears (2, peeled, seeded, quartered)

Lime (1, juiced)

Water (2 cups)

Directions:

Add all your ingredients into your blender, and blend.

Set a fine mesh strainer a bowl. Before transferring your juice into the strainer.

Gently press the pulp to extract all possible liquid then discard pulp.

Serve over ice. Enjoy!

Nutrition:

247 calories, 1 g fat, 65 g carbs, 10 g fiber, 3 g protein

45. Pineapple Ice Cubes

Preparation Time: 4 hrs. 10 mins.

Cooking Time: 0 mins.

Servings: 24 ice cubes

Ingredients:

Pineapple Juice (3 cups, unsweetened).

Directions:

Fill your empty ice trays with your juice.

Set to freeze for at least 3 hours until frozen.

Transfer your flavored ice cubes to freezer bags.

Keep them in the freezer until ready to serve.

Nutrition:

70 calories, 0 g fat, 18 g carbs, 2 g fiber, 1 g protein

46. Gala Apple Flavored Ice Cubes

Preparation Time: 4 hrs. 10 mins.

Cooking Time: 0 mins.

Servings: 24 ice cubes

Ingredients:

Apple (2, Gala)

Honey (4 tsp.)

Water (3 cups)

Directions:

Add all your ingredients into your blender, and blend.

Set a fine mesh strainer a bowl. Before transferring your juice into the strainer.

Gently press the pulp to extract all possible liquid then discard pulp.

Fill your empty ice trays with your juice.

Set to freeze for at least 3 hours until frozen.

Transfer your flavored ice cubes to freezer bags.

Keep them in the freezer until ready to serve.

Nutrition:

83 calories,1 g fat, 21 g carbs, 2 g fiber, 1 g protein

47. Kale Flavored Ice Cubes

Preparation Time: 4 hrs. 10 mins.

Cooking Time: 0 mins.

Servings: 24 ice cubes

Ingredients:

Honey (¼ cup)

Water (2 cups)

Kale (3 cups, chopped)

Directions:

Add all your ingredients into your blender, and blend.

Set a fine mesh strainer a bowl. Before transferring your juice into the strainer.

Gently press the pulp to extract all possible liquid then discard pulp.

Fill your empty ice trays with your juice.

Set to freeze for at least 3 hours until frozen.

Transfer your flavored ice cubes to freezer bags.

Keep them in the freezer until ready to serve.

Nutrition:

110 calories, 1 g fat, 25 g carbs, 4 g fiber, 3 g protein

48.   Cranberry Flavored Ice Cubes

Preparation Time: 4 hrs. 10 mins.

Cooking Time: 0 mins.

Servings: 24 ice cubes

Ingredients:

Cranberry Juice (3 cups, unsweetened)

Directions:

Fill your empty ice trays with your juice.

Set to freeze for at least 3 hours until frozen.

Transfer your flavored ice cubes to freezer bags.

Keep them in the freezer until ready to serve.

Nutrition:

120 calories, 2 g fat, 24g carbs, 1 g fiber, 0 g protein

49.   Banana Ice Cubes

Preparation Time: 15 mins.

Cooking Time: 0 mins.

Servings: 24 ice cubes

Ingredients:

Bananas (2, peeled, sliced)

Honey (1 tbsp.)

Water (3 cups)

Directions:

Add all your ingredients into your blender, and blend.

Set a fine mesh strainer a bowl. Before transferring your juice into the strainer.

Gently press the pulp to extract all possible liquid then discard pulp.

Fill your empty ice trays with your juice.

Set to freeze for at least 3 hours until frozen.

Transfer your flavored ice cubes to freezer bags.

Keep them in the freezer until ready to serve.

Nutrition:

71 calories, 0 g fat, 16 g carbs, 1 g fiber, 2 g protein

## 50.	Elderberry Gummies

Preparation Time: 7 mins.

Cooking Time: 4 hrs.

Servings: 20-50

Ingredients:

Gelatin (2 tbsp.)

Water (1/4 cup, room temperature)

Hot Water (1/4 cup)

Orange Juice (1/2 cup)

Lemon Juice (2 tbsp.)

Elderberry Soothing Syrup (2 tbsp.)

Directions:

Combine your gelatin and room temperature water, stirring until fully dissolved.

Stir in your hot water then leave to rest for about 2 minutes.

Add in your remaining ingredients and stir until combined.

Transfer to serving size containers then place on a tray in the refrigerator to set for about 4 hours.

Enjoy!

Nutrition:

3 calories, 0 g fat, 1 g carbs, 0 g fiber, 0 g protein

51.   Blackberry-Rose Ice Pops

Preparation Time: 25 mins.

Cooking Time: 5 hrs.

Servings: 10

Ingredients:

cane sugar (9 tbsp., organic)

Water (9 tbsp., for simple syrup)

blackberries (6 1/2 cups)

lemon juice (1 tbsp.)

rosewater (1 tsp.)

Water (1 cup)

Directions:

Create a simple syrup by heating sugar and the water for the simple syrup over medium heat.

Allow the mixture to simmer, stirring until the sugar dissolves. Set to cool (about 10 minutes).

Add all your ingredients into your blender, and blend.

Set a fine mesh strainer a bowl. Before transferring your juice into the strainer.

Gently press the pulp to extract all possible liquid then discard pulp.

Pour your juice into your ice-pop molds, filling each three quarters of the way.

Add in your ice pop sticks then set to freeze for at least 5 hours or until solid.

Unmold and enjoy.

Nutrition:

112 calories, 0 g fat, 30g carbs, 5 g fiber, 1 g protein

52.   Frozen Strawberry-Peach Pops

Preparation Time: 5 mins.

Cooking Time: 0 mins.

Servings: 5

Ingredients:

Sugar (1/2 cup)

Strawberries (6 oz.)

Peaches (6 oz.)

Water (4 oz.)

Lemon Juice (1 tbsp.)

Directions:

Create a simple syrup by heating sugar and water over medium heat.

Allow the mixture to simmer, stirring until the sugar dissolves. Set to cool (about 10 minutes).

Add all your ingredients into your blender, and blend.

Set a fine mesh strainer a bowl. Before transferring your juice into the strainer.

Gently press the pulp to extract all possible liquid then discard pulp.

Pour your juice into your ice-pop molds, filling each three quarters of the way.

Add in your ice pop sticks then set to freeze for at least 5 hours or until solid. Unmold and enjoy.

Nutrition:

102 calories, 1 g fat, 12g carbs, 2 g fiber,2 g protein

53.   Honey Lemonade Popsicles

Preparation Time: 5 mins.

Cooking Time: 0 mins.

Servings: 8

Ingredients:

Honey (1/2 cup)

Lemon Juice (12 oz.)

Water (6 oz.)

Directions:

Create honey water by heating honey and over medium heat.

Allow the mixture to simmer, stirring until the honey melts. Set to cool (about 10 minutes).

In a spouted container, combine all your ingredients.

Pour your juice into your ice-pop molds, filling each three quarters of the way.

Add in your ice pop sticks then set to freeze for at least 5 hours or until solid. Unmold and enjoy.

Nutrition:

36 calories, 3 g fat, 3 g carbs, 1g fiber, 3 g protein

54.   Orange Strawberry Popsicles

Preparation Time: 10 mins.

Cooking Time: 0 mins.

Servings: 12 popsicles

Ingredients:

Strawberry (4 cups, hulled)

orange juice (2 cups)

lime (1, juiced)

Honey (1/4 cup)

Directions:

Add all your ingredients into your blender, and blend.

Set a fine mesh strainer a bowl. Before transferring your juice into the strainer.

Gently press the pulp to extract all possible liquid then discard pulp.

Pour your juice into your ice-pop molds, filling each three quarters of the way.

Nutrition:

160 calories, 0 g fat, 40 g carbs, 1 g fiber, 0 g protein

55. Melon Basil Moscow Mule Popsicles

Preparation Time: 5 mins.

Cooking Time: 0 mins.

Servings: 10 popsicles

Ingredients:

Cantaloupe (1 lb., peeled, seeded chopped)

Mint (7 leaves)

Water (4 oz.)

Limeade (4 oz.)

Ginger Beer (16 oz.)

Simple Syrup (2 oz.)

Directions:

Add all your ingredients into your blender, and blend.

Set a fine mesh strainer a bowl. Before transferring your juice into the strainer.

Gently press the pulp to extract all possible liquid then discard pulp.

Pour your juice into your ice-pop molds, filling each three quarters of the way.

Nutrition:

34 calories, 0 g fat, 8 g carbs, 1 g fiber, 2 g protein

56.   Honeydew Mint Homemade Popsicles

Preparation Time: 10 mins.

Cooking Time: 0 mins.

Servings: 10 popsicles

Ingredients:

Honeydew melon (1/2, peeled, cubed)

Granulated sugar (1/3 cup)

Mint (10 leaves)

Lime juice (1 tbsp.)

Water (6 oz.)

xanthan gum (1 pinch)

Directions:

Add all your ingredients into your blender, and blend.

Set a fine mesh strainer a bowl. Before transferring your juice into the strainer.

Gently press the pulp to extract all possible liquid then discard pulp.

Pour your juice into your ice-pop molds, filling each three quarters of the way.

Nutrition:

34 calories, 0 g fat, 8 g carbs, 1 g fiber, 2 g protein

57.   Raspberry Lemonade Popsicles

Preparation Time: 5 mins.

Cooking Time: 0 mins.

Servings: 10 popsicle

Ingredients:

lemonade concentrate (2 cup)

lemon-lime soda (48 oz.)

Fresh raspberries (1 pint)

Directions:

Add all your ingredients into your blender, and blend.

Set a fine mesh strainer a bowl. Before transferring your juice into the strainer.

Gently press the pulp to extract all possible liquid then discard pulp.

Pour your juice into your ice-pop molds, filling each three quarters of the way.

Nutrition:

43 calories, 1 g fat, 6 g carbs, 1 g fiber, 4 g protein

58.   Strawberry Popsicles

Preparation Time: 10 mins.

Cooking Time: 0 mins.

Servings: 12 popsicle

Ingredients:

Strawberries (4 cups, hulled)

Water (2 cups)

Lime (1, juiced)

Honey (1/4 cup)

Directions:

Create a simple syrup by heating sugar and water over medium heat.

Allow the mixture to simmer, stirring until the sugar dissolves. Set to cool (about 10 minutes).

Add all your ingredients into your blender, and blend.

Set a fine mesh strainer a bowl. Before transferring your juice into the strainer.

Gently press the pulp to extract all possible liquid then discard pulp.

Pour your juice into your ice-pop molds, filling each three quarters of the way.

Nutrition:

60 calories, 1 g fat, 15 g carbs, 1 g fiber, 2 g protein

59.   Basil Watermelon Popsicles

Preparation Time: 10 mins.

Cooking Time: 0 mins.

Servings: 12 popsicle

Ingredients:

Watermelon (1 lb.)

Basil (5 leaves)

Water (12 oz.)

Lime Juice (4 oz.)

Honey (1 oz.)

Directions:

Create honey water by heating honey and over medium heat.

Allow the mixture to simmer, stirring until the honey melts. Set to cool (about 10 minutes).

In a spouted container, combine all your ingredients.

Pour your juice into your ice-pop molds, filling each three quarters of the way.

Add in your ice pop sticks then set to freeze for at least 5 hours or until solid. Unmold and enjoy.

Nutrition:

47 calories, 0 g fat, 12 g carbs, 1 g fiber, 1 g protein

60.   Orange Popsicles

Preparation Time: 10 mins.

Cooking Time: 0 mins.

Servings: 12 popsicle

Ingredients:

orange juice (3 cups)

lime (1, juiced)

Directions:

Set a fine mesh strainer a bowl. Before transferring your juice into the strainer.

Gently press the pulp to extract all possible liquid then discard pulp.

Pour your juice into your ice-pop molds, filling each three quarters of the way.

Nutrition:

121 calories, 0 g fat,12 g carbs, 1 g fiber, 0 g protein

61.   Grapefruit Lemonade Popsicles

Preparation Time: 10 mins.

Cooking Time: 0 mins.

Servings: 8 popsicle

Ingredients:

Honey (1/4 cup)

Grapefruit Juice (2½ cup)

Lemon Juice (12 oz.)

Water (6 oz.)

Directions:

Create honey water by heating honey and over medium heat.

Allow the mixture to simmer, stirring until the honey melts. Set to cool (about 10 minutes).

In a spouted container, combine all your ingredients.

Pour your juice into your ice-pop molds, filling each three quarters of the way.

Add in your ice pop sticks then set to freeze for at least 5 hours or until solid. Unmold and enjoy.

Nutrition:

71 calories, 0.1 g fat, 17.3 g carbs, 0.1 g fiber, 0.3 g protein

## 62.	Ginger Beer Gelatin Dessert

Preparation Time: 5 mins.

Cooking Time: 3 hrs.

Servings: 8 serving

Ingredients:

Raspberries (2 cups, chopped)

Water (1 cup)

Gelatin (2 tbsp.)

Ginger Beer (1 1/2 cups)

Lemon Juice (1 tbsp.)

Stevia to taste, if desired

Directions:

Stir your gelatin into your water then set it to rest in a saucepan for about 5 minutes.

Set to heat up on low heat until glossy and lump free.

Combine all your remaining ingredients then slowly stir in your gelatin mix.

Transfer to molds then set to refrigerate for about 4 hours or until set. Enjoy!

Nutrition:

67 calories, 0 g fat, 6 g carbs, 1 g fiber, 1 g protein

Chapter 5. Low Fiber Recipes

Breakfast

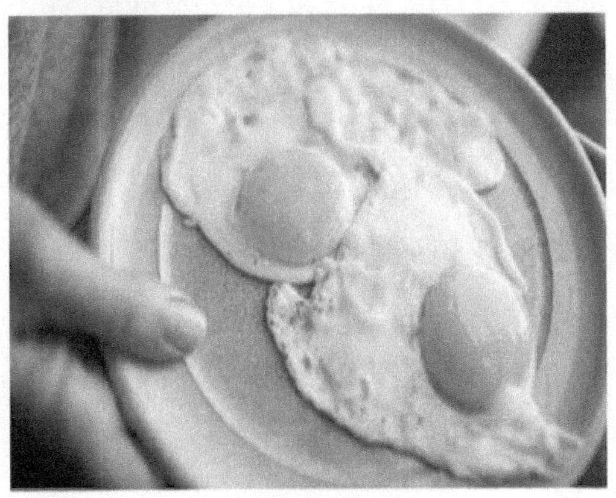

63. Oatmeal Waffles

Preparation Time: 10 mins.

Cooking Time: 15 mins.

Servings: 2-3

Ingredients:

Quick Oats (1 1/2 cups)

White flour (1/2 cup, refined)

baking powder (1 tbs)

cinnamon (1 tbs)

nutmeg (1 tsp)

egg (1)

banana (1, mashed)

honey (1 tbs)

milk (1 1/2 cups)

cooking spray (Non-stick)

Directions:

In a large bowl mix together oatmeal, cinnamon, baking powder, whole wheat flour, and nutmeg. Set aside.

In a separate bowl, mix egg, banana, honey, and milk. Mix dry mixture into wet mixture. Preheat waffle iron.

Spray with non-stick cooking spray.

Pour less than 1/4 cup batter into hot pan for each waffle.

Cook until puffy and dry around edges. Turn and cook other side until golden.

Nutrition:

404 calories, 7 g fat, 47 g carbs, 6 g fiber, 15 g protein

64. Spinach Frittata

Preparation Time: 10 mins.

Cooking Time: 30 mins.

Servings: 4

Ingredients:

olive oil (2 tsp)

red pepper (1 cup, seeded, chopped)

garlic (1 clove, minced)

spinach leaves (3 cups, chopped)

eggs (4, large, beaten)

salt (1/2 tsp)

Parmesan cheese (1/4 cup, freshly grated)

Directions:

Preheat oven to 350 degrees. In a non-stick oven pan, heat 1 tsp olive oil over medium heat.

Cook red peppers and garlic until vegetables are soft (about 10 minutes). In medium bowl, combine eggs and spinach and salt; set aside.

Add remaining 1 tsp olive oil into pan with vegetables and add in the egg mixture.

Turn the heat to medium and cook for 15 mins. Sprinkle Parmesan cheese over top of mixture and broil for an additional 4 minutes.

Nutrition:

106 calories, 8 g fat, 7 g carbs, 2 g fiber, 3 g protein

65. Banana and Pear Pita Pockets

Preparation Time: 5 mins.

Cooking Time: 25 mins.

Servings: 1

Ingredients:

Banana (1/2 small, peeled, sliced)

pita bread (1, round, made with refined white flour)

pear (1/2, small, peeled, seedless, cored, cooked, sliced)

cottage cheese (1/4 cup, low fat

Directions:

Combine banana, pear, and cottage cheese in a small bowl. Slice pita to make a pocket. Fill pita pocket with mixture. Serve.

Nutrition:

402 calories, 2 g fat, 87 g carbs, 11 g fiber, 14 g protein

66. Pear Pancakes

Preparation Time: 5 mins.

Cooking Time: 15 mins.

Servings: 4

Ingredients:

Eggs (2)

Pear (1 cup, peeled mashed)

Cinnamon (1 tsp)

Sugar (2 tsp)

Refined white flour (1 1/2 cup)

flour (1/2 cup, whole-wheat)

baking powder (2 tsp)

vanilla (2 tsp)

cooking spray (Non-stick)

Directions:

In a medium bowl, beat eggs until fluffy. Add baking powder, cinnamon, vanilla, sugar, flours, and pear, and continue to stir just until smooth. Heat griddle or non-stick pan over medium heat.

Spray with non-stick cooking spray. Pour a sizeable amount of batter that you want your pancake to be into the hot pan.

Cook pancakes until puffy and dry around edges. Turn and cook other side until golden. Serve pancakes with additional pear if desired.

Nutrition:

174 calories, 2 g fat, 34 g carbs, 2 g fiber, 5 g protein

67. Ripe Plantain Bran Muffins

Preparation Time: 10 mins.

Cooking Time: 20 mins.

Servings: 12

Ingredients:

Refined Cereal (1 1/2 cups)

Milk (2/3 cup, low fat)

Eggs (4, large, lightly beaten)

canola oil (1/4 cup)

ripe plantain (2, medium, mashed, 1 cup)

brown sugar (1/2 cup)

refined flour (1 cup, white)

baking powder (2 tsp)

salt (1/2 tsp)

Directions:

Preheat oven to 400F degrees. In a large bowl, combine bran cereal and milk and set aside.

Add eggs and oil; stir in brown sugar and mashed ripe plantain. In another bowl, combine salt, flour, and baking powder.

Add the dry ingredients into the ripe plantain mixture, stir until combined.

Pour batter evenly into a paper-lined muffin tins; Bake 18 minutes or until golden-brown and firm. Allow to cool prior to serving.

Nutrition:

325 calories, 19 g fat, 37 g carbs, 2 g fiber, 3 g protein

68.   Easy Breakfast Bran Muffins

Preparation Time: 10 mins.

Cooking Time: 20 mins.

Servings: 10

Ingredients:

Refined cereal (2 cups)

brown sugar (1/2 cup)

butter (1/2 cup)

eggs (2)

buttermilk (1/2 quart)

white flour (2 1/2 cups, refined)

baking soda (2 1/2 tsp)

salt (1/2 tsp)

Directions:

Preheat oven to 400F degrees. Soak 1 cup cereal in 1 cup boiling water and set aside.

In a mixer, cream sugar and butter together until it is fully mixed. Add each egg separate and beat until fluffy. Add buttermilk and soaked cereal mixture.

In another bowl, combine salt, flour and baking soda. Add the flour mixture into the batter and ensure not to over mix.

Add in remaining 1 cup of cereal. Pour batter evenly into 10 greased or paper-lined muffin tins. Bake 15-20 minutes. Allow to cool prior to serving.

Nutrition:

440 calories, 20 g fat, 57 g carbs, 3 g fiber, 9 g protein

69.   Apple Oatmeal

Preparation Time: 8 mins.

Cooking Time: 1mins.

Servings: 1

Ingredients:

Instant oatmeal (1/2 cup)

milk or water (3/4 cup)

apples (1/2 cup, peeled, cooked pureed)

brown sugar (1 tsp)

Directions:

In a microwave-safe bowl, mix oats, milk or water and apples. Cook in microwave on high for 45 seconds.

Stir and microwave for another 30 seconds. Sprinkle with brown sugar and add a splash of milk.

Nutrition:

295 calories, 7 g fat, 47 g carbs, 5 g fiber, 13 g protein

70.   Breakfast Burrito Wrap

Preparation Time: 15 mins.

Cooking Time: 15 mins.

Servings: 1

Ingredients:

olive oil (1 tbs, extra virgin)

turkey bacon (2 slices)

green bell peppers (1/4 cup, seeded and chopped)

eggs (2, beaten)

milk (2 tbs)

salt (1/4 tsp)

Monterrey Jack cheese (2 tbs, low- fat, grated)

Tortilla (1, white)

Directions:

In a small non-stick pan, heat olive oil on medium heat and cook turkey about 2 minutes until slightly crispy.

Add bell peppers and continue to cook until warmed through. In a small bowl beat together egg with milk and salt.

Gently stir in your eggs until almost cooked through. Turn the heat down then add the cheese.

Cover and continue to cook until cheese have completely melted. Place the mixture on the tortilla and roll it into a burrito.

Nutrition:

355 calories, 2 g fat, 14 g carbs, 4 g fiber, 23 g protein

71.   Zucchini Omelet

Preparation Time: 15 mins.

Cooking Time: 15 mins.

Servings: 4

Ingredients:

olive oil (2 tbs, extra virgin)

zucchini (1, medium, seeded, cubed)

tomato (1/2 medium, seeded, chopped)

eggs (4, large)

milk (1/4 cup)

salt (1 tsp)

English muffins (4, whole wheat)

Directions:

In a large non-stick pan, heat olive oil over moderate heat. Add zucchini and tomato.

Cook vegetables for 5-10 minutes or until they are soft. In a separate bowl, mix eggs and milk and salt.

Add egg mixture to pan and stir to cook through, about 5 minutes. Serve with white English muffins.

Nutrition:

160 calories, 10 g fat, 14 g carbs, 2 g fiber, 6 g protein

72. Coconut Chia Seed Pudding

Preparation Time: 10 mins.

Cooking Time: 0 mins.

Servings: 2

Ingredients:

chia seeds (6 tbsp.)

coconut milk (2 cups, unsweetened)

Blueberries for topping

Directions:

Combine the chia seeds and milk and mix well. Refrigerate overnight. Stir in the berries and serve.

Nutrition:

223 calories, 12 g fat, 18 g carbs, 2 g fiber, 10 g protein

73. Spiced Oatmeal

Preparation Time: 5 mins.

Cooking Time: 2 mins.

Servings: 1

Ingredients:

quick oats (1/3 cup)

banana (1/2)

ginger (1/4 tsp., ground)

cinnamon (1/8 tsp., ground)

small sprinkle nutmeg ground

small sprinkle cloves ground

1 tbsp. almond butter

Directions:

Combine the oats and water. Microwave for 45 seconds, then stir and cook for another 30-45 seconds.

Stir in the spices and drizzle on the almond butter before serving.

Nutrition:

467 calories, 11 g fat, 33 g carbs, 4 g fiber, 6 g protein

74. Breakfast Cereal

Preparation Time: 5 mins.

Cooking Time: 5 mins.

Servings: 4

Ingredients:

old fashioned oatmeal (3 cups, cooked)

quinoa (3 cups, cooked)

4 cups banana, peeled, chopped

Directions:

Combine the oatmeal and quinoa and mix well. Evenly divide into four bowls and top with the bananas before serving.

Nutrition:

228 calories, 3 g fat, 43 g carbs, 6 g fiber, 12 g protein

75.   Sweet Potato Hash with Sausage & Spinach

Preparation Time: 5 mins.

Cooking Time: 15 mins.

Servings: 4

Ingredients:

sweet potatoes (4 small, chopped)

apples (2, cored and chopped)

1 clove garlic (minced)

sausage (1 lb., ground)

spinach (10 oz chopped)

Salt & pepper

Directions:

Brown the sausage until no pink remains. Add the remaining ingredients.

Cook for an additional 5-6 minutes, or until the spinach and apples are tender. Season to taste and serve hot.

Nutrition:

544 calories, 2 g fat, 65 g carbs, 2 g fiber, 11 g protein

76.   Cajun Omelet

Preparation Time: 5 mins.

Cooking Time: 8 mins.

Servings: 2

Ingredients:

sausage (1/4 lb., spicy)

mushrooms (1/3 cup, sliced)

onion (1/2, diced eggs (4 large)

½ medium bell pepper, chopped

water (2 tbsp.)

cooking Fat

1 pinch cayenne pepper (optional)

Sea salt & fresh pepper to taste

Directions:

Brown the sausage in a medium saucepan until cooked through. Add the mushrooms, onion and bell pepper and cook for another3-5 minutes, or until tender.

Meanwhile, whisk together the eggs, water, mustard and spices. Season with the salt and pepper.

Top with your eggs over then reduce to a low heat. Cook until the top is nearly set and then fold the omelet in half and cover. Cook for another minute before serving hot.

Nutrition:

467 calories, 14 g fat, 11 g carbs, 2 g fiber, 3 g protein

77.   **Strawberry Cashew Chia Pudding**

Preparation Time: 10 mins.

Cooking Time: 0 mins.

Servings: 2

Ingredients:

chia seeds (6 tbsp.)

cashew milk (2 cups, unsweetened)

Strawberries, for topping

Directions:

Combine the chia seeds and milk and mix well. Refrigerate overnight. Stir in the berries and serve.

Nutrition:

223 calories, 12 g fat, 18 g carbs, 2 g fiber, 10 g protein

78.   Peanut Butter Banana Oatmeal

Preparation Time: 5 mins.

Cooking Time: 5 mins.

Servings: 1

Ingredients:

quick oats (1/3 cup)

cinnamon (1/4 tsp. (optional)

banana (1/2, sliced)

peanut butter (1 tbsp., unsweetened)

Directions:

Combine all ingredients in a bowl with a lid. Refrigerate.

Nutrition:

645 calories, 32g fat, 65 g carbs, 5 g fiber, 26g protein

79.   Asparagus Frittata

Preparation Time: 15 minutes

Cooking Time: 20 minutes

Servings: 4

Ingredients

½ cup of sliced shallots

2 tablespoons of unsalted butter

½ teaspoon of salt

6 large eggs

A pound thin spear asparagus. The tough ends should be snapped off, and cut into lengths of one inch each

¾ cup of ricotta cheese

A cup of shredded Swiss cheese or Gruyere cheese

¼ teaspoon of dried tarragon.

Directions:

First, you have to cook the shallots in butter. To do this, you heat the butter in a frying pan. Heat over medium-heat.

Place the shallots in the heated butter and cook. Stir intermittently while cooking until they become soft and translucent. This should take about 3 minutes.

Next, throw in the asparagus and cook for an extra three minutes.

Prepare an egg mix. To do this, you beat the ricotta cheese and eggs together, then add salt, tarragon, and chives. Put the egg mixture in the pan and cook for 4-5 minutes, or until it is almost set. Preheat the oven broiler while the egg mixture is cooking.

Sprinkle the cheese over the eggs and broil in the oven until the cheese melts and browns, and the center sets. This should take between 6-8 minutes.

Wearing your oven mitts, take the pan out of the oven and put the frittata on serving plates. Cut into wedges.

80. Chicken Pasta Salad

Preparation Time: 10 minutes

Cooking time: 20 minutes

Servings: 8

Ingredients

Salad

1 lb. of fusilli pasta

One teaspoon of garlic powder

A pound of boneless skinless chicken breasts

Kosher salt

A tablespoon of extra-virgin olive oil

2c halved grape tomatoes

4 slices of bacon, should be cooked and crumbled

2c of spinach, packed

¼ red onion, sliced thinly

2 tablespoons of freshly chopped dill

Crumbled feta – 1/2c

Dressing

3 tablespoon of red wine vinegar

1/4c extra-virgin olive oil

1 clove garlic, minced

½ teaspoon of Italian seasoning

Kosher salt

1 tablespoon of Dijon mustard

Freshly ground black pepper

Directions:

Put some salt in a large pot of water and boil it. Cook the fusilli in the boiling water according to instructions on the packaging. Drain and turn into a large bowl.

Season the chicken breasts with salt, pepper, and garlic powder. Heat some oil over medium heat in a large skillet. Cook the chicken breast until it becomes golden. Cook each side for 8 minutes.

Allow the cooked chicken to rest for 8 minutes, then cut into pieces of 1 inch each.

Prepare the dressing. Here's how to do it: whisk oil, Italian seasoning, vinegar, mustard, garlic. Season with pepper and salt.

Toss the pasta with the rest of the ingredients in a large bowl. Spread the dressing over the salad, toss until it coats well, then serve.

81.   Roasted Beet Salad With Goat Cheese

Preparation Time: 15 minutes

Cooking Time: 45 minutes

Servings: 4

Ingredients

¼ cup of chopped walnuts

¼ cup of pomegranate arils

¼ cup of goat cheese

1 teaspoon of Dijon mustard

2 teaspoons of pure maple syrup

½ cup of pomegranate juice

2 teaspoons of minced shallot

A pound of beets

1/8 teaspoon of kosher salt, and some extra for roasting

Black pepper for roasting and seasoning

5 ounces of baby arugula

2 teaspoons of apple cider vinegar

¾ cup of extra virgin olive oil

Directions:

Place the oven rack in the center and preheat to 204oC.

Trim the top of the beets. Allow ½ inch of the stem. Wash and dry.

Place the beets on a large foil. Coat the beets with olive oil, then sprinkle with pepper and salt. Wrap tightly in the foil and put on a sheet tray.

Roast the beets until they are tender. This should take between 40 to 60 minutes. Of course, the time spent cooking will depend on the size of the beets. Check for doneness every 20 minutes.

Leave the beets to cool, then peel, cut into wedges of ½ inch, and set aside.

Add apple cider, pomegranate juice, maple syrup, mustard, and shallots, to a blender. Blend at medium speed until it smoothens. This will take up to 15 seconds.

Add ¾ cups of olive oil to the running blender. When adding the oil, do it slowly until the dressing becomes thick. Season with pepper and 1/8 teaspoon of salt.

Serve topped with goat cheese, sliced beets, chopped walnuts, and pomegranate arils.

Serve with pomegranate dressing.

Use a countertop blender for this.

82. Zucchini & Onions With Veggie Omelette

Preparation Time: 10 minutes

Cooking Time: 10 minutes

Servings: 2

Ingredients

2 tablespoons of flat-leaf parsley (minced)

¼ tablespoon of ground pepper

2 egg whites

¾ teaspoon of olive oil

3 eggs

¼ teaspoon of salt

A tablespoon of crumbled feta cheese

3 tablespoons of water

¼ cup of grated zucchini

1/3 cup of chopped onion

How to prepare

Start by heating the olive oil in a skillet set over medium heat.

Cook the onion, stirring intermittently, until they begin to brown. This should take up to 4 minutes.

Next, throw in the grated zucchini and cook for 120 seconds. After cooking, turn the vegetables into a plate. Cover the plate with the foil to keep them warm.

Whisk the eggs in a medium bowl together with water and egg whites. Whisk until they are well-combined.

Clean your skillet and coat with cooking spray. Then raise the heat to medium-high.

Cook the eggs in the skillet until their edges set. Lift the edge of the omelet gently using a spatula then slightly tilt the pan so that the uncooked egg mixture can run to the bottom of the pan. Do this continually as the egg cooks.

When the center is set, you season with pepper and salt.

Scoop the vegetable mixture onto one-half of the omelet. Top with feta cheese.

Loosen the omelet with a spatula, then fold in half. Place on a cutting board and cut in half, then serve.

Best garnished with parsley.

Nutrition:

Sugar 2g | Fiber 0.9g | Potassium 273.3mg | Sodium 356.2mg | Cholesterol 282.3mg | Saturated fat 3.2g | Fat 9.8g | Protein 14g | Carbohydrates 4.1g | Calories 162.8kcal

83.   Banana Bran Muffins

Preparation Time: 10 minutes

Cooking Time: 25 minutes

Servings: 12

Ingredients

½ cup of brown sugar

½ cup of butter, softened

¼ cup of milk

2 large eggs

3 medium bananas (mashed)

11/2 cups of all-purpose flour

½ cup of wheat bran

A teaspoon of baking soda

A teaspoon of baking powder

½ cup of chopped walnuts

¼ teaspoon of salt

Preparation

Preheat your oven to 1900C. Line a muffin pan with paper muffin liners, or you may grease it.

Cream brown sugar and butter in a large mixing bowl until they become fluffy. Add milk, eggs, vanilla, and bananas. Mix thoroughly, then stir in the bran, flour, soda, baking powder, and salt. Blend until it becomes moist. Stir in the walnuts. Pour the batter into the muffin cups.

Bake for 20-25 minutes at 1900C. To be sure that it is done, dip a toothpick into the center of the muffin. If it comes out clean, then it is done. Allow it to cool in the cups for 5 minutes, then take out the muffins and cool it off completely on a rack.

Nutrition:

Sodium: 265.5mg | cholesterol: 51.7mg | fat: 12.2g | Carbohydrates: 30.4g | Protein: 4.4g | Calories: 239

84.   Peach Oatmeal

Preparation Time: 5 minutes

Cooking Time: 0 minutes

Servings: 3

Ingredients

A cup of milk

2 cups of old fashioned oats

¾ teaspoon of vanilla extract

A tablespoon of brown sugar

¼ cup of granola – best for garnishing

¼ teaspoon of ground nutmeg

½ teaspoon of ground cinnamon

½ cup of peach slices

Preparation

Stir milk and oats in a medium bowl

Microwave for 90 seconds or until the oats soften

Add the sugar (or honey), vanilla, nutmeg, and cinnamon. Stir and fold in peaches.

Spoon the oatmeal into two bowls and garnish with peach slices. Top with some granola and enjoy!

Nutrition:

Iron: 3mg| Calcium: 133mg| Vitamin C: 2mg| Vitamin A: 215IU| Sugar: 13g| Fiber: 7g| Potassium: 391mg| Sodium: 43mg| Cholesterol: 8mg| Saturated fat: 2g| Fat: 8g| Protein: 11g| Carbohydrates: 54g| Calories: 332 kcal

Lunch

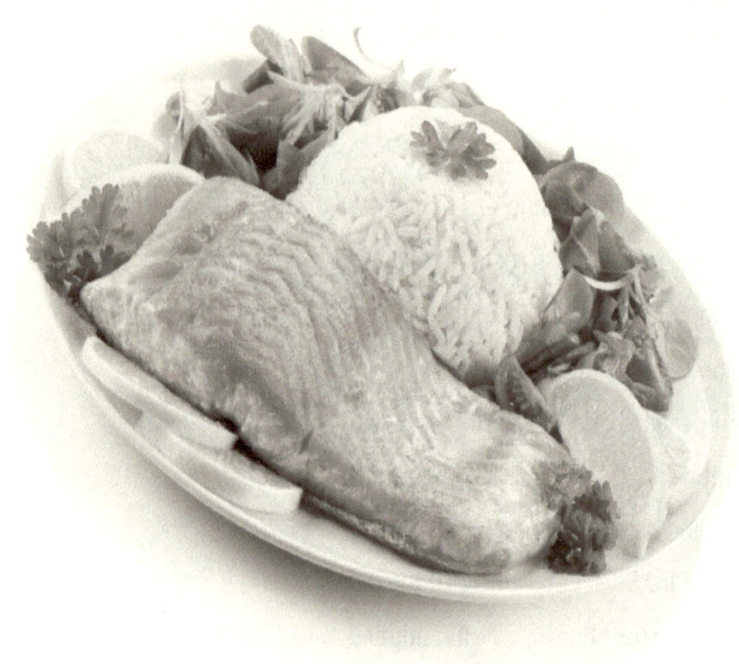

85.　　Super-Food Scramble

Preparation Time: 10 minutes

Cooking Time: 7 minutes

Servings: 3

Ingredients:

2 C. fresh spinach, chopped finely

1 tbsp. olive oil

Salt and freshly ground black pepper, to taste

½ C. cooked salmon, chopped finely

4 eggs, beaten

Directions:

In a skillet, heat the oil over high heat and cook the spinach with black pepper for about 2 minutes.

Stir in the salmon and reduce the heat to medium.

Add the eggs and cook for about 3-4 minutes, stirring frequently.

Serve immediately.

Nutrition:

Calories per serving: 179; Carbohydrates: 1.2g; Protein: 15.3g; Fat: 12.9g; Sugar: 0.5g; Sodium: 165mg; Fiber: 0.4g

86.   Family Favorite Scramble

Preparation Time: 10 minutes

Cooking Time: 5 minutes

Servings: 2

Ingredients:

4 eggs

¼ tsp. red pepper flakes, crushed

Salt and freshly ground black pepper, to taste

¼ C. fresh basil, chopped

½ C. tomatoes, peeled, seeded and chopped

1 tbsp. olive oil

Directions:

In a large bowl, add eggs, red pepper flakes, salt and black pepper and beat well.

Add the basil and tomatoes and stir to combine.

In a large non-stick skillet, heat the oil over medium-high heat.

Add the egg mixture and cook for about 3-5 minutes, stirring continuously.

Serve immediately.

Nutrition:

Calories per serving: 195; Carbohydrates: 2.6g; Protein: 11.6g; Fat: 15.9g; Sugar: 1.9g; Sodium: 203mg; Fiber: 0.7g

87.   **Tasty Veggie Omelet**

Preparation Time: 15 minutes

Cooking Time: 25 minutes

Servings: 4

Ingredients:

6 large eggs

Sea salt and freshly ground black pepper, to taste

½ C. low-fat milk

1/3 C. fresh mushrooms, cut into slices

1/3 C. red bell pepper, seeded and chopped

1 tbsp. chives, minced

Directions:

Preheat the oven to 350 degrees F. Lightly, grease a pie dish.

In a bowl, add the eggs, salt, black pepper and coconut oil and beat until well combined.

In another bowl, mix together the onion, bell pepper and mushrooms.

Transfer the egg mixture into the prepared pie dish evenly.

Top with vegetable mixture evenly and sprinkle with chives evenly.

Bake for about 20-25 minutes.

Remove from the oven and set aside for about 5 minutes.

With a knife, cut into equal sized wedges and serve.

Nutrition:

Calories per serving: 125; Carbohydrates: 3.1g; Protein: 10.8g; Fat: 7.8g; Sugar: 2.8g; Sodium: 158mg; Fiber: 0.2g

88.   **Garden Veggies Quiche**

Preparation Time: 15 minutes

Cooking Time: 20 minutes

Servings: 4

Ingredients:

6 eggs

½ C. low-fat milk

Salt and freshly ground black pepper, to taste

2 C. fresh baby spinach, chopped

½ C. green bell pepper, seeded and chopped

1 scallion, chopped

¼ C. fresh parsley, chopped

1 tbsp. fresh chives, minced

Directions:

Preheat the oven to 400 degrees F. Lightly grease a pie dish.

In a bowl, add eggs, almond milk, salt and black pepper and beat until well combined. Set aside.

In another bowl, add the vegetables and herbs and mix well.

In the bottom of prepared pie dish, place the veggie mixture evenly and top with the egg mixture.

Bake for about 20 minutes or until a wooden skewer inserted in the center comes out clean.

Remove pie dish from the oven and set aside for about 5 minutes before slicing.

Cut into desired sized wedges and serve warm.

Nutrition:

Calories per serving: 118; Carbohydrates: 4.3g; Protein: 10.1g; Fat: 7g; Sugar: 3g; Sodium: 160mg; Fiber: 0.8g

89. Fluffy Pumpkin Pancakes

Preparation Time: 10 minutes

Cooking Time: 40 minutes

Servings: 10

Ingredients:

2 eggs

1 C. buckwheat flour

1 tbsp. baking powder

1 tsp. pumpkin pie spice

½ tsp. salt

1 C. pumpkin puree

¾ C. plus 2 tbsp. low-fat milk

3 tbsp. pure maple syrup

2 tbsp. olive oil

1 tsp. vanilla extract

Directions:

In a blender, add all ingredients and pulse until well combined.

Transfer the mixture into a bowl and set aside for about 10 minutes.

Heat a greased non-stick skillet over medium heat.

Place about ¼ C. of the mixture and spread in an even circle.

Cook for about 2 minutes per side.

Repeat with the remaining mixture.

Serve warm.

Nutrition:

Calories per serving: 113; Carbohydrates: 16.5g; Protein: 3.6g; Fat: 4.4g; Sugar: 5.9g; Sodium: 143mg; Fiber: 2g

## 90.	Sper-Tasty Chicken Muffins

Preparation Time: 15 minutes

Cooking Time: 45 minutes

Servings: 8

Ingredients:

8 eggs

Salt and freshly ground black pepper, as required

2 tbsp. filtered water

7 oz. cooked chicken, chopped finely

1½ C. fresh spinach, chopped

1 C. green bell pepper, seeded and chopped finely

2 tbsp. fresh parsley, chopped finely

Directions:

Preheat the oven to 350 degrees F. Grease 8 C. of a muffin tin.

In a bowl, add eggs, salt, black pepper and water and beat until well combined.

Add the chicken, spinach, bell pepper and parsley and stir to combine.

Transfer the mixture into the prepared muffin C. evenly.

Bake for about 18-20 minutes or until golden brown.

Remove the muffin tin from oven and place onto a wire rack to cool for about 10 minutes.

Carefully invert the muffins onto a platter and serve warm.

Nutrition:

Calories per serving: 107; Carbohydrates: 1.7g; Protein: 13.1g; Fat: 5.2g; Sugar: 1.1g; Sodium: 102mg; Fiber: 0.4g

91. Classic Zucchini Bread

Preparation Time: 45 minutes

Cooking Time: 15 minutes

Servings: 24

Ingredients:

3 C. all-purpose flour

2 tsp. baking soda

1 tsp. ground cinnamon

1 tsp. ground nutmeg

2 C. Splenda

1 C. olive oil

3 eggs, beaten

2 tsp. vanilla extract

2 C. zucchini, peeled, seeded and grated

Directions:

Preheat the oven to 325 degrees F. Arrange a rack in the center of oven. Grease 2 loaf pans.

In a medium bowl, mix together the flour, baking soda and spices.

In another large bowl, add the Splenda and oil and beat until well combined.

Add the eggs and vanilla extract and beat until well combined.

Add the flour mixture and mix until just combined.

Gently, fold in the zucchini.

Place the mixture into the bread loaf pans evenly.

Bake for about 45-50 minutes or until a toothpick inserted in the center of bread comes out clean.

Remove the bread pans from oven and place onto a wire rack to cool for about 15 minutes.

Carefully, invert the breads onto the wire rack to cool completely before slicing.

With a sharp knife, cut each bread loaf into desired-sized slices and serve.

Nutrition:

Calories per serving: 219; Carbohydrates: 28.4g; Protein: 16.3g; Fat: 9.2g; Sugar: 16.3g; Sodium: 113mg; Fiber: 0.6g

92.   Greek Inspired Cucumber Salad

Preparation Time: 10 minutes

Cooking Time: 0 minutes

Servings: 4

Ingredients:

4 medium cucumbers, peeled, seeded and chopped

½ C. low-fat Greek yogurt

1½ tbsp. fresh dill, chopped

1 tbsp. fresh lemon juice

Salt and freshly ground black pepper, as required

Directions:

In a large bowl, add all the ingredients and mix well.

Serve immediately.

Nutrition:

Calories per serving: 71; Carbohydrates: 13.8g; Protein:4g; Fat: 0.8g; Sugar: 7.3g; Sodium: 69mg; Fiber: 1.7g

93.   Light Veggie Salad

Preparation Time: 10 minutes

Cooking Time: 0 minutes

Servings: 5

Ingredients:

2 C. cucumbers, peeled, seeded and chopped

2 C. red tomatoes, peeled, seeded and chopped

2 tbsp. extra-virgin olive oil

2 tbsp. fresh lime juice

Salt, to taste

Directions:

In a large serving bowl, add all the ingredients and toss to coat well.

Serve immediately.

Nutrition:

Calories per serving: 68; Carbohydrates: 04.4g; Protein: 0.9g; Fat: 5.8g; Sugar: 2.6g; Sodium: 35mg; Fiber: 1.1g

94. Eastern European Soup

Cooking Time: 5 minutes

Preparation Time: 10 minutes

Servings: 3

Ingredients:

2 C. fat-free yogurt

4 tsp. fresh lemon juice

2 C. beets, trimmed, peeled and chopped

2 tbsp. fresh dill

Salt, as required

1 tbsp. fresh chives, minced

Directions:

In a high-speed blender, add all ingredients except for chives and pulse until smooth.

Transfer the soup into a pan over medium heat and cook for about 3-5 minutes or until heated through.

Serve immediately with the garnishing of chives.

Nutrition:

Calories per serving: 149; Carbohydrates: 25.2g; Protein: 11.8g; Fat: 0.6g; Sugar: 21.7g; Sodium: 269mg; Fiber: 2.5g

95. Citrus Glazed Carrots

Preparation Time: 15 minutes

Cooking Time: 15 minutes

Servings: 6

Ingredients:

1½ lb. carrots, peeled and sliced into ½-inch pieces diagonally

½ C. water

2 tbsp. olive oil

Salt, to taste

3 tbsp. fresh orange juice

Directions:

In a large skillet, add the carrots, water, boil and salt over medium heat and bring to a boil.

Reduce heat to low and simmer; covered for about 6 minutes.

Add the orange juice and stir to combine.

Increase the heat to high and cook, uncovered for about 5-8 minutes, tossing frequently.

Serve immediately.

Nutrition:

Calories per serving: 90; Carbohydrates: 12g; Protein: 1g; Fat: 4.7g; Sugar: 6.2g; Sodium: 106mg; Fiber: 2.8g

96.   Braised Asparagus

Preparation Time: 10 minutes

Cooking Time: 8 minutes

Servings: 2

Ingredients:

½ C. chicken bone broth

1 tbsp. olive oil

1 (½-inch) lemon peel

1 C. asparagus, trimmed

Directions:

In a small pan add the broth, oil and lemon peel over medium heat and bring to a boil.

Add the asparagus and cook, covered for about 3-4 minutes.

Discard the lemon peel and serve.

Nutrition:

Calories per serving: 82; Carbohydrates: 2.6g; Protein: 3.7g; Fat: 7.1g; Sugar: 1.3g; Sodium: 25mg; Fiber: 1.4g

97. Spring Flavored Pasta

Preparation Time: 10 minutes

Cooking Time: 10 minutes

Servings: 4

Ingredients:

2 tbsp. olive oil

1 lb. asparagus, trimmed and cut into 1½-inch pieces

Salt and freshly ground black pepper, to taste

½ lb. cooked hot pasta, drained

Directions:

In a large cast-iron skillet, heat the oil over medium heat and cook the asparagus, salt and black pepper for about 8-10 minutes, stirring occasionally.

Place the hot pasta and toss to coat well.

Serve immediately.

Nutrition:

Calories per serving: 246 Carbohydrates: 35.2g; Protein: 8.9g; Fat: 8.4g; Sugar: 2.1g; Sodium: 17mg; Fiber: 2.4g

98.   Versatile Mac 'n Cheese

Preparation Time: 15 minutes

Cooking Time: 12 minutes

Servings: 1

Ingredients:

2 C. elbow macaroni

1½ s butternut squash, peeled and cubed

1 C. low-fat Swiss cheese, shredded

1/3 C. low-fat milk

1 tbsp. olive oil

Salt and freshly ground black pepper, to taste

Directions:

In a large pan of the salted boiling water, cook the macaroni for about 8-10 minutes.

Drain the macaroni and transfer into a bowl.

Meanwhile, in a pan of the boiling water, cook the squash cubes for about 6 minutes or until soft.

Drain the squash cubes completely and return to the same pan.

With a masher, mash the squash and place over low heat.

Add the cheese and milk and cook for about 2-3 minutes, stirring continuously.

Add the macaroni, oil, salt and black pepper and stir to combine.

Remove from the heat and serve hot.

Nutrition:

Calories per serving: 321; Carbohydrates: 40g; Protein: 14g; Fat: 11.9g; Sugar: 3.7g; Sodium: 65mg; Fiber: 2.4g

99.   Gluten-Free Curry

Preparation Time: 15 minutes

Cooking Time: 20 minutes

Servings: 6

Ingredients:

2 C. tomatoes, peeled, seeded and chopped

1½ C. water

2 tbsp. olive oil

1 tsp. fresh ginger, chopped

¼ tsp. ground turmeric

2 C. fresh shiitake mushrooms, sliced

5 C. fresh button mushrooms, sliced

¼ C. fat-free yogurt, whipped

Salt and freshly ground black pepper, to taste

Directions:

In a food processor, add the tomatoes and ¼ C. of water and pulse until a smooth paste forms.

In a pan, heat the oil over medium heat and sauté the ginger and turmeric for about 1 minute.

Add the tomato paste and cook for about 5 minutes.

Stir in the mushrooms, yogurt and remaining water and bring to a boil.

Cook for about 10-12 minutes, stirring occasionally.

Season with the salt and black pepper and remove from the heat.

Serve hot.

Nutrition:

Calories per serving: 70; Carbohydrates: 5.3g; Protein: 3g; Fat: 5g; Sugar: 3.4g; Sodium: 41mg; Fiber: 1.4g

100.   New Year's Luncheon Meal

Preparation Time: 10 minutes

Cooking Time: 0 minutes

Servings: 2

Ingredients:

1 large avocado, halved and pitted

1 (5-oz.) can water-packed tuna, drained and flaked

3 tbsp. fat-free yogurt

2 tbsp. fresh lemon juice

1 tsp. fresh parsley, chopped finely

Salt and freshly ground black pepper, to taste

Directions:

Carefully, remove abut about 2-3 tbsp. of flesh from each avocado half.

Arrange the avocado halves onto a platter and drizzle each with 1 tsp. of lemon juice.

Chop the avocado flesh and transfer into a bowl.

In the bowl of avocado flesh, add tuna, yogurt, parsley, remaining lemon juice, salt, and black pepper, and stir to combine.

Divide the tuna mixture in both avocado halves evenly.

Serve immediately.

Nutrition:

Calories per serving: 215; Carbohydrates: 7g; Protein: 20.6g; Fat: 11.8g; Sugar: 2.4g; Sodium: 137mg; Fiber: 3.2g

101. Entertaining Wraps

Preparation Time: 15 minutes

Cooking Time: 10 minutes

Servings: 5

Ingredients:

For Chicken:

2 tbsp. olive oil

1 tsp. fresh ginger, minced

1¼ lb. ground chicken

Salt and freshly ground black pepper, to taste

For Wraps:

10 romaine lettuce leaves

1½ C. carrot, peeled and julienned

2 tbsp. fresh parsley, chopped finely

2 tbsp. fresh lime juice

Directions:

In a skillet, heat the oil over medium heat and sauté the ginger for about 1 minute.

Add the ground chicken, salt, and black pepper and cook for about 7-9 minutes, breaking up the meat into smaller pieces with a wooden spoon.

Remove from the heat and set aside to cool.

Arrange the lettuce leaves onto serving plates.

Place the cooked chicken over each lettuce leaf and top with carrot and cilantro.

Drizzle with lime juice and serve immediately.

Nutrition:

Calories per serving: 280; Carbohydrates: 3.8g; Protein: 33.2g; Fat: 14g; Sugar: 1.7g; Sodium: 153mg; Fiber: 0.9g

Snack

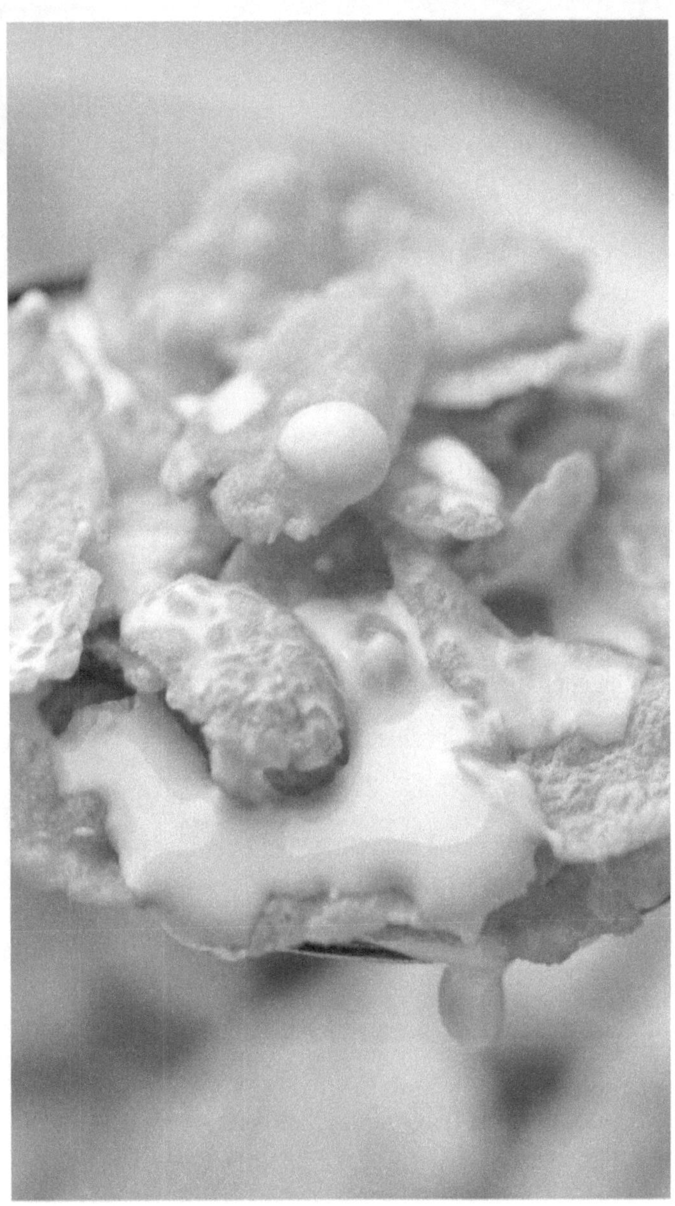

102.   Almond Peanut Butter Fudge

Preparation Time: 2 hrs.10 mins.

Cooking Time: 0 mins.

Servings: 2

Ingredients:

peanut butter (1 cup, unsweetened)

vanilla almond milk (1/4 cup, unsweetened)

coconut oil (1 cup)

vanilla liquid stevia (2 tsps., optional)

Salt - pinch

For the Chocolate Sauce (topping):

melted coconut oil (2 tbsps.)

cocoa powder (1/4 cup, unsweetened)

maple syrup (2 tbsps.)

Directions:

For Chocolate Sauce:

Take a bowl and add the coconut oil, maple syrup and cocoa powder

Whisk together completely and keep it aside.

For Peanut Butter Fudge:

Slightly melt the coconut oil and peanut butter together over low heat on the stove (you can also use the microwave).

Add this melted mixture, vanilla almond milk, stevia and salt to the blender. Blend well until thoroughly combined.

Pour this blended mixture to a loaf pan lined with a parchment. Refrigerate for 2 hours until set.

Drizzle the chocolate sauce over the fudge after it has been set. Refrigerate it for some more time and then serve.

Nutrition:

287calories, 30 g fat, 4 g carbs, 2g fiber, 5 g protein

103.   Quick Cocoa Mousse

Preparation Time: 10 mins.

Cooking Time: 0 mins.

Servings: 8

Ingredients:

heavy whipping cream (6 tbsps., whip it and keep ready)

butter (4 tbsps., unsalted)

cocoa powder (1 tbsp)

cream cheese (4 tbsps.)

coconut oil (1 tsp)

Stevia (as per taste)

Directions:

Soften the butter in a microwave and then combine it with stevia. Stir well until it blends completely.

Add the cream cheese and cocoa powder to the butter mixture. Blend thoroughly until it becomes smooth.

Slowly add the whipped heavy cream to the mixture and keep stirring. Add 1 tsp of MCT oil or coconut oil to the mixture and blend again.

Spoon the smooth mixture into small glasses and refrigerate for 30 minutes. Serve chilled.

Nutrition:

227 calories, 2 g fat, 3 g carbs, 1 g fiber, 4 g protein

104. Cinnamon Pear Chips

Preparation Time: 5 mins.

Cooking Time: 3 hrs.

Servings: 4

Ingredients:

Pears (4)

ground cinnamon (1 teaspoon)

Directions:

Preheat the oven to 200°F. Line a baking sheet with parchment paper.

Core the pears and cut into 1/8-inch slices. Toss pears with cinnamon.

Spread the pears in a single layer on the prepared baking sheet. Cook for 2 to 3 hours, until the pears are dry.

They will still be soft while hot but will crisp once completely cooled. Store in an airtight container for up to four days.

Nutrition:

96 calories, 0 g fat, 26 g carbs, 1 g fiber, 1 g protein

105.   Chocolate Yogurt Cream & Roasted Bananas

Preparation Time: 10 mins.

Cooking Time: 5 mins.

Servings: 4

Ingredients:

whipping cream (½ cup)

ground cinnamon (½ tsp)

low fat vanilla yogurt (1 ½ cups, chilled and drained)

cold butter (1 tbsp)

confectioner's sugar (1 tbsp)

dark rum (1 tbsp)

unsweetened cocoa powder (2 tbsp)

dark brown sugar (3 tbsp)

bananas (4, cut in strips)

Directions:

Place bananas cut side up on a baking sheet coated with cooking spray.

Sprinkle with brown sugar, rum and cinnamon. Dot with butter.

Roast in a 425-degree Fahrenheit preheated oven for five minutes. Turn the broiler off until the bananas are golden.

Meanwhile, beat the cocoa, cream and confectioner's sugar in a large bowl using an electric mixer.

Add the drained yogurt and fold the cream until well combined. Plate the roasted bananas and add a dollop of chocolate cream on top.

Nutrition:

236 calories, 0 g fat, 42g carbs, 3 g fiber, 7 g protein

106.   Coconut Celery Smoothie

Preparation Time: 10 mins.

Cooking Time: 0 mins.

Servings: 2

Ingredients:

celery stalks (3, shredded)

ground cinnamon (1 tsp)

banana (½)

protein powder (1 scoop)

coconut butter (1 tbsp)

unsweetened coconut milk (1 cup)

Directions:

Toss your ingredients into a blender then process until creamy and smooth. Serve immediately and enjoy.

Nutrition:

391 calories, 15 g fat, 42 g carbs, 1 g fiber, 29 g protein

107.   Apple Spinach Smoothie

Preparation Time: 10 mins.

Cooking Time: 0 mins.

Servings: 2

Ingredients:

vanilla extract (¼ tsp)

ginger (1 tsp, grated)

maple syrup (1 tsp)

coconut butter (1 ½ tbsp)

yogurt (½ cup)

apple (1, chopped)

baby spinach (1 cup)

unsweetened coconut milk (1 cup)

Directions:

Toss your ingredients into a blender then process until creamy and smooth. Serve immediately and enjoy.

Nutrition:

388 calories, 19 g fat, 43 g carbs, 3 g fiber, 15 g protein

Dinner

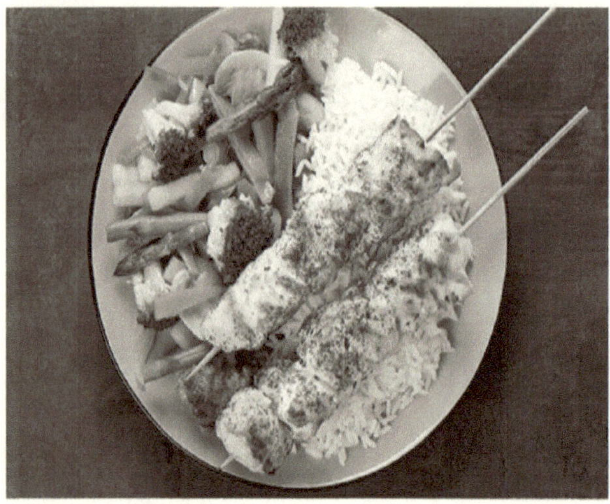

108. **Outdoor Chicken Kabobs**

Preparation Time: 15 minutes

Cooking Time: 7 minutes

Servings: 4

Ingredients:

¼ C. low-fat Parmesan cheese, grated

3 tbsp. olive oil

1 C. fresh basil leaves, chopped

Salt and freshly ground black pepper, to taste

1¼ lb. boneless, skinless chicken breast, cut into 1-inch cubes

Directions:

In a food processor, add the cheese, oil, garlic, basil, salt, and black pepper, and pulse until smooth.

Transfer the basil mixture into a large bowl.

Add the chicken cubes and mix well.

Cover the bowl and refrigerate to marinate for at least 4-5 hours.

Preheat the grill to medium-high heat. Generously, grease the grill grate.

Thread the chicken cubes onto pre-soaked wooden skewers.

Place the skewers onto the grill and cook for about 3-4 minutes.

Flip and cook for about 2-3 minutes more.

Remove from the grill and place onto a platter for about 5 minutes before serving.

Serve hot.

Nutrition:

Calories per serving: 270; Carbohydrates: 0.3g; Protein: 31.5g; Fat: 15.3g; Sugar: 0g; Sodium: 207mg; Fiber: 0.1g

109. Flavorful Shrimp Kabobs

Preparation Time: 15 minutes

Cooking Time: 8 minutes

Servings: 4

Ingredients:

¼ C. olive oil

2 tbsp. fresh lime juice

1 tsp. honey

½ tsp. paprika

¼ tsp. ground cumin

Salt and freshly ground black pepper, to taste

1 lb. medium raw shrimp, peeled and deveined

Directions:

In a large bowl, add all the ingredients except for shrimp and mix well.

Add the shrimp and coat with the herb mixture generously.

Refrigerate to marinate for at least 30 minutes.

Preheat the grill to medium-high heat. Grease the grill grate.

Thread the shrimp onto pre-soaked wooden skewers.

Place the skewers onto the grill and cook for about 2-4 minutes per side.

Remove from the grill and place onto a platter for about 5 minutes before serving.

Nutrition:

Calories per serving: 250; Carbohydrates: 3.4g; Protein: 25.9g; Fat: 14.6g; Sugar: 01.5g; Sodium: 316mg; Fiber: 0.1g

110.   Pan-Seared Scallops

Preparation Time: 15 minutes

Cooking Time: 7 minutes

Servings: 4

Ingredients:

1¼ lb. fresh sea scallops, side muscles removed

Salt and freshly ground black pepper, to taste

2 tbsp. olive oil

1 tbsp. fresh parsley, minced

Directions:

Sprinkle the scallops with salt and black pepper.

In a large skillet, heat the oil over medium-high heat and cook the scallops for about 2-3 minutes per side.

Stir in the parsley and remove from the heat.

Serve hot.

Nutrition:

Calories per serving: 185; Carbohydrates: 3.4g; Protein: 23.8g; Fat: 8.1g; Sugar: 0g; Sodium: 268mg; Fiber: 0g

111. Mediteranean Shrimp Salad

Preparation Time: 15 minutes

Cooking Time: 3 minutes

Servings: 5

Ingredients:

1 lb. shrimp, peeled and deveined

1 lemon, quartered

2 tbsp. olive oil

2 tsp. fresh lemon juice

Salt and freshly ground black pepper, to taste

3 tomatoes, peeled, seeded and sliced

¼ C. olives, pitted

¼ C. fresh cilantro, chopped finely

Directions:

In a pan of the lightly salted water, add the quartered lemon and bring to a boil.

Add the shrimp and cook for about 2-3 minutes or until pink and opaque.

With a slotted spoon, transfer the shrimp into a bowl of ice water to stop the cooking process.

Drain the shrimp completely and then pat dry with paper towels.

In a small bowl, add the oil, lemon juice, salt, and black pepper, and beat until well combined.

Divide the shrimp, tomato, olives, and cilantro onto serving plates.

Drizzle with oil mixture and serve.

Nutrition:

Calories per serving: 178; Carbohydrates: 5g; Protein: 21.4g; Fat: 8g; Sugar: 2.1g; Sodium: 315mg; Fiber: 1.2g

112.   Helth Conscious People's Salad

Preparation Time: 15 minutes

Cooking Time: 0 minutes

Servings: 2

Ingredients:

¼ C. low-fat mozzarella cheese, cubed

¼ C. tomato, peeled, seeded and chopped

1 tbsp. fresh dill, chopped

1 tsp. fresh lemon juice

Salt, to taste

6 oz. cooked salmon, chopped

Directions:

In a small bowl, add all the ingredients and stir to combine.

Serve immediately.

Nutrition:

Calories per serving: 131; Carbohydrates: 1.9g; Protein: 18g; Fat: 6g; Sugar: 0.6g; Sodium: 141mg; Fiber: 0.5g

113. Italian Pasta Soup

Cooking Time: 25 minutes

Preparation Time: 15 minutes

Servings: 5

Ingredients:

1 potato, peeled and chopped

1 carrot, peeled and chopped

5¼ C. chicken bone broth

½ C. tomato, peeled, seeded and chopped

¾ lb. asparagus tips

½ C. cooked small pasta

Salt and freshly ground black pepper, to taste

Directions:

In a pan, add the potato, carrot and broth over medium-high heat and bring to a boil.

Reduce the heat to low and cook, covered for about 15 minutes or until vegetables become tender.

Add the tomatoes and asparagus and cook or about 4-5 minutes.

Stir in the cooked pasta, salt and black pepper and cook for about 2-3 minutes.

Serve hot.

Nutrition:

Calories per serving: 147; Carbohydrates: 23.2g; Protein: 13.6g; Fat: 0.5g; Sugar: 3.5g; Sodium: 108mg; Fiber: 3g

114. Pure Comfort Soup

Cooking Time: 20 minutes

Preparation Time: 10 minutes

Servings: 4

Ingredients:

6 C. chicken bone broth

1/3 C. orzo

6 large egg yolks

1½ C. cooked chicken, shredded

¼ C. fresh lemon juice

Salt and freshly ground black pepper, to taste

Directions:

In a large pan, add the broth over medium-high heat and bring to a boil.

Add the pasta and cook for about 8-9 minutes.

In a slowly, add in 1 C. of the hot broth, beating continuously.

Add the egg mixture to the pan, stirring continuously.

Reduce the heat to medium and cook for about 5-7 minutes, stirring, frequently.

Stir in the cooked chicken, salt and black pepper and cook for about 1-2 minutes.

Remove from the heat and serve hot.

Nutrition:

Calories per serving: 269; Carbohydrates: 11.9g; Protein: 34.6g; Fat: 8.7g; Sugar: 1.2g; Sodium: 230mg; Fiber: 0.6g

115.   Goof-for-You Stew

Cooking Time: 18 minutes

Preparation Time: 15 minutes

Servings: 8

Ingredients:

2½ C. fresh tomatoes, peeled, seeded and chopped

4 C. fish bone broth

1 lb. salmon fillets, cubed

1 lb. shrimp, peeled and deveined

2 tbsp. fresh lime juice

Salt and freshly ground black pepper, to taste

3 tbsp. fresh parsley, chopped

Directions:

In a large soup pan, add the tomatoes and broth and bring to a boil.

Reduce the heat to medium and simmer for about 5 minutes.

Add the salmon and simmer for about 3-4 minutes.

Stir in the shrimp and cook for about 4-5 minutes.

Stir in lemon juice, salt, and black pepper, and remove from heat.

Serve hot with the garnishing of parsley.

Nutrition:

Calories per serving: 173; Carbohydrates: 3.2g; Protein: 27.1g; Fat: 5.5g; Sugar: 1.5g; Sodium: 368mg; Fiber: 0.7g

116.   Zero-Fiber Chicken Dish

Cooking Time: 10 minutes

Preparation Time: 16 minutes

Servings: 6

Ingredients:

4 (6-oz.) boneless, skinless chicken breast halves

Salt and freshly ground black pepper, to taste

2 tbsp. olive oil

Directions:

Season each chicken breast half with salt and black pepper evenly.

Place chicken breast halves over a rack set in a rimmed baking sheet.

Refrigerate for at least 30 minutes.

Remove from refrigerator and pat dry with paper towels.

In a skillet, heat the oil over medium-low heat.

Place the chicken breast halves, smooth-side down, and cook for about 9-10 minutes, without moving.

Flip the chicken breasts and cook for about 6 minutes or until cooked through.

Remove from the heat and let the chicken stand in the pan for about 3 minutes.

Now, place the chicken breasts onto a cutting board.

Cut each chicken breast into slices and serve.

Nutrition:

Calories per serving: 255; Carbohydrates: 0g; Protein: 32.8g; Fat: 13.1g; Sugar: 0g; Sodium: 125mg; Fiber: 0g

117.   Amazing Chicken Platter

Cooking Time: 18 minutes

Preparation Time: 15 minutes

Servings: 6

Ingredients:

2 tbsp. olive oil, divided

4 (4-oz.) boneless, skinless chicken breasts, cut into small pieces

Salt and freshly ground black pepper, to taste

1 tsp. fresh ginger, grated

4 C. fresh mushrooms, sliced

1 C. chicken bone broth

Directions:

In a large skillet, heat 1 tbsp. of oil over medium-high heat and stir fry the chicken pieces, salt, and black pepper for about 4-5 minutes or until golden-brown.

With a slotted spoon, transfer the chicken pieces onto a plate.

In the same skillet, heat the remaining oil over medium heat and sauté the onion, ginger for about 1 minute.

Add the mushrooms and cook for about 6-7 minutes, stirring frequently.

Add the cooked chicken and coconut milk and stir fry for about 3-4 minutes

Add in the salt and black pepper and remove from the heat.

Serve hot.

Nutrition:

Calories per serving: 200; Carbohydrates: 1.6g; Protein: 24.8g; Fat: 10.4g; Sugar: 0.8g; Sodium: 111mg; Fiber: 0.5g

118.   Colorful Chicken Dinner

Cooking Time: 20 minutes

Preparation Time: 15 minutes

Servings: 6

Ingredients:

3 tbsp. olive oil, divided

1 large yellow bell pepper, seeded and sliced

1 large red bell pepper, seeded and sliced

1 large green bell pepper, seeded and sliced

1 lb. boneless, skinless chicken breasts, sliced thinly

1 tsp. dried oregano, crushed

¼ tsp. garlic powder

¼ tsp. ground cumin

Salt and freshly ground black pepper, to taste

¼ C. chicken bone broth

Directions:

In a skillet, heat 1 tbsp. of oil over medium-high heat and cook the bell peppers for about 4-5 minutes.

With a slotted spoon, transfer the peppers mixture onto a plate.

In the same skillet, heat the remaining over medium-high heat and cook the chicken for about 8 minutes, stirring frequently.

Stir in the thyme, spices, salt, black pepper, and broth, and bring to a boil.

Add the peppers mixture and stir to combine.

Reduce the heat to medium and cook for about 3-5 minutes or until all the liquid is absorbed, stirring occasionally.

Serve immediately.

Nutrition:

Calories per serving: 226; Carbohydrates: 4.8g; Protein: 22.9g; Fat: 12.8g; Sugar: 3g; Sodium: 98mg; Fiber: 0.9g

119.　Easiest Tuna Salad

Preparation Time: 15 minutes

Cooking Time: 0 minutes

Ingredients:

Servings: 4

For Dressing:

2 tbsp. fresh dill, minced

2 tbsp. olive oil

1 tbsp. fresh lime juice

Salt and freshly ground black pepper, to taste

For Salad:

2 (6-oz.) cans water-packed tuna, drained and flaked

6 hard-boiled eggs, peeled and sliced

1 C. tomato, peeled, seeded and chopped

1 large cucumber, peeled, seeded and sliced

Directions:

For dressing: in a small bowl, add all the ingredients and beat until well combined.

For salad: in another large serving bowl, add all the ingredients and mix well.

Divide the tuna mixture onto serving plates.

Drizzle with dressing and serve.

Nutrition:

Calories per serving: 277; Carbohydrates: 5.9g; Protein: 31.2g; Fat: 14.5g; Sugar: 3g; Sodium: 181mg; Fiber: 1.1g

120.   Lemony Salmon

Preparation Time: 10 minutes

Cooking Time: 14 minutes

Servings: 4

Ingredients:

1 tbsp. fresh lemon zest, grated

2 tbsp. extra-virgin olive oil

2 tbsp. fresh lemon juice

Salt and freshly ground black pepper, to taste

4 (6-oz.) boneless, skinless salmon fillets

Directions:

Preheat the grill to medium-high heat. Grease the grill grate.

In a bowl, place all ingredients except for salmon fillets and mix well.

Add the salmon fillets and coat with garlic mixture generously.

Place the salmon fillets onto grill and cook for about 6-7 minutes per side.

Serve hot.

Nutrition:

Calories per serving: 290; Carbohydrates: 1g; Protein: 33.2g; Fat: 21.5g; Sugar: 0.3g; Sodium: 116mg; Fiber: 0.2g

121.   Herbed Salmon

Cooking Time: 8 minutes

Preparation Time: 10 minutes

Servings: 4

Ingredients:

1 tsp. dried oregano, crushed

1 tsp. dried basil, crushed

Salt and freshly ground black pepper, to taste

¼ C. olive oil

2 tbsp. fresh lemon juice

4 (4-oz.) salmon fillets

Directions:

In a large bowl, add all ingredients except for salmon and mix well.

Add the salmon and coat with marinade generously.

Cover the bowl and refrigerate to marinate for at least 1 hour.

Preheat the grill to medium-high heat. Grease the grill grate.

Place the salmon onto the grill and cook for about 4 minutes per side.

Serve hot.

Nutrition:

Calories per serving: 261; Carbohydrates: 0.4g; Protein: 22.1g; Fat: 19.7g; Sugar: 0.2g; Sodium: 80mg; Fiber: 0.2g

122.   Delicious Combo Dinner

Preparation Time: 15 minutes

Cooking Time: 15 minutes

Servings: 5

Ingredients:

2 tbsp. olive oil

1 lb. prawns, peeled and deveined

1 lb. asparagus, trimmed

Salt and freshly ground black pepper, to taste

1 tsp. fresh ginger, minced

2 tbsp. fresh lemon juice

Directions:

In a skillet, heat 1 tbsp. of oil over medium-high heat and cook the prawns with salt and black pepper for about 3-4 minutes.

With a slotted spoon, transfer the prawns into a bowl. Set aside.

In the same skillet, heat the remaining oil over medium-high heat and cook the asparagus, ginger, salt and black pepper for about 6-8 minutes, stirring frequently.

Stir in the prawns and cook for about 1 minute.

Stir in the lemon juice and remove from the heat.

Serve hot.

Nutrition:

Calories per serving: 176; Carbohydrates: 5.1g; Protein: 22.7g; Fat: 7.3g; Sugar: 1.9g; Sodium: 255mg; Fiber: 1.9g

Dessert

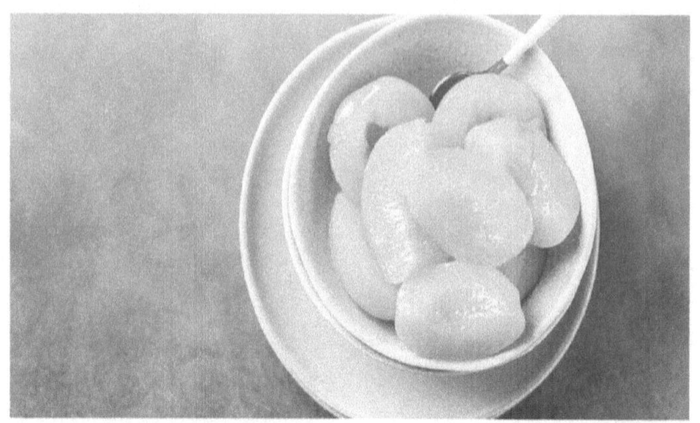

123. Banana Cocoa Cream

Preparation Time: 4 hrs.

Cooking Time: 0 mins.

Servings: 4

Ingredients:

Banana (1, mashed)

cocoa powder, to taste

stevia, to taste (optional)

Directions:

Mix one mashed banana with stevia and cocoa powder. You may blend these together or use a food processor for best results.

Freeze in a sealed container for 2-4 hours.

Nutrition:

0.1 calories, 1 g fat, 7 g carbs, 1g fiber, 0 g protein

124. Homemade Pumpkin Pie

Preparation Time: 5 mins.

Servings: 10

Cooking Time: 45 mins.

Ingredients:

Crust:

1, half-batch All Butter Pie crust, fitted into a 9-inch, crimped and chilled

Filling:

pumpkin purée (1, 15- ounce, can)

sugar (¾ cup)

eggs (2 large, at room temperature)

lactose-free evaporated milk (11- ounces)

cinnamon (1 teaspoon)

ginger (½ teaspoon, ground)

salt (1/4 teaspoon)

cloves (¼ teaspoon, ground)

Directions:

Position rack in center of oven. Set oven to preheat to 425°F. Whisk eggs, sugar and pumpkin together in medium bowl.

Whisk in your salt, cinnamon, ginger, clove and evaporated milk until smooth.

Add filling to your crust and set to bake for 15 minutes. Turn heat down to 350°F (180°C) and continue to bake until filling is set, about 35 to 45 minutes.

Cool completely then serve. Pie is best served the day it is baked but it can be made 1 day ahead; store at room temperature lightly covered with foil.

Nutrition:

342 calories, 1 g fat, 42 g carbs, 1 g fiber, 5 g protein

125. Chocolate Pear Cream

Preparation Time: 4 hrs.

Cooking Time: 0 mins.

Servings: 4

Ingredients:

Pear (1, cooked, mashed)

cocoa powder, to taste

stevia, to taste (optional)

Directions:

Mix one mashed pear with stevia and cocoa powder.

You may blend these together or use a food processor for best results. Freeze in a sealed container for 2-4 hours.

Nutrition:

96 calories, 1 g fat, 7 g carbs, 1 g fiber, 0g protein

126.   Zero Sugar Pumpkin Pie

Preparation Time: 10 mins.

Cooking Time: 1 hr.

Servings: 16

Ingredients:

Pumpkin (1 15oz can)

ground cinnamon (3/4 tsp.)

ground nutmeg (1/2 tsp.)

ground ginger (1/2 tsp)

ground cloves (1/2 tsp.)

Evaporated Skim Milk (1 14oz can)

Eggs (2 large, slightly beaten)

Splenda (1/2 cup)

Pie Crust (9" deep dish, refined white flour)

Directions:

Baked at 350 degrees for 1 hour. Makes 16 small servings.

Nutrition:

84 calories, 3 g fat, 1 g carbs, 3 g fiber, 35 g protein

127. Orange Curd

Preparation Time:5 mins.

Cooking Time:15 mins.

Servings: 20

Ingredients:

Butter (55g)

Sugar (225g)

Eggs (2 Large, beaten)

Juice and finely grated zest of 2 oranges

Directions:

Put a bowl over a pan of simmering water and add the butter and sugar until dissolved. Add the orange zest and juice.

Gently whisk while adding the eggs. Let it cook gently stirring until it is thick and like custard this should take 15 minutes. Remove it from the heat and place it into a jar.

Nutrition:

72 calories, 3 g fat, 12 g carbs, 1g fiber, 1 g protein

128. Instant Pot Pear Crumble

Preparation Time: 15 mins.

Cooking Time: 25 mins.

Servings: 6

Ingredients:

pears (5 large, cut into 1-inch chunks)

water (1/3 cup)

flour (3 Tbsp)

quick oats (¾ cup)

coconut sugar (½ cup)

ground cinnamon (2 tsp)

fine sea salt (¼ tsp)

melted coconut oil or butter (¼ cup)

Directions:

Add your water and pears into your Instant Pot and stir well to be sure the pears cover the bottom of the pot in an even layer.

In a separate bowl, combine salt, cinnamon, sugar, oats and flour then stir well.

Add the melted coconut oil and stir until thoroughly mixed. Top pears with crumble.

Select Manual/Pressure. Cook on high pressure for 8 minutes. Naturally release the pressure from your IP (about 10 minutes).

Remove the lid. Use oven mitts to remove the dish from the Instant Pot and let the crumble cool for 10 minutes before serving warm.

Nutrition:

279 calories, 10 g fat, 48 g carbs, 1 g fiber, 2 g protein

129.   Sweet Potato Cream Pie

Preparation Time: 5 mins.

Cooking Time: 16 mins.

Servings: 4

Ingredients:

water (1 cup)

sweet potato (1, peeled and diced)

coconut milk (½ cup full-fat canned)

pure maple syrup (6 Tbsp, plus more as needed)

fresh ginger (1 tsp, grated, about ½-inch knob)

Directions:

Add 1 cup water to the Instant Pot and arrange a steamer basket on the bottom. Place the sweet potato pieces in the steamer basket and cover.

Seal your steam valve. Set the IP on Pressure Cook or Manual mode then cook on High for 10 minutes.

When ready, immediately move the steam release valve to Venting to quickly release the steam pressure.

Use oven mitts to lift the steamer basket out of the pot and transfer the cooked potatoes to a large bowl.

Add the coconut milk, maple syrup, and ginger. Use an immersion blender or potato masher to puree the potatoes into a smooth pudding.

Taste and adjust the flavor, adding more ginger or maple syrup as needed. Serve the pudding right away, or chill it in the fridge.

Store leftover pudding in an airtight container in the fridge for 1 week.

Nutrition:

181 calories, 2 g fat, 18g carbs, 0g fiber, 35 g protein

Chapter 6. High Fiber Recipes

Breakfast

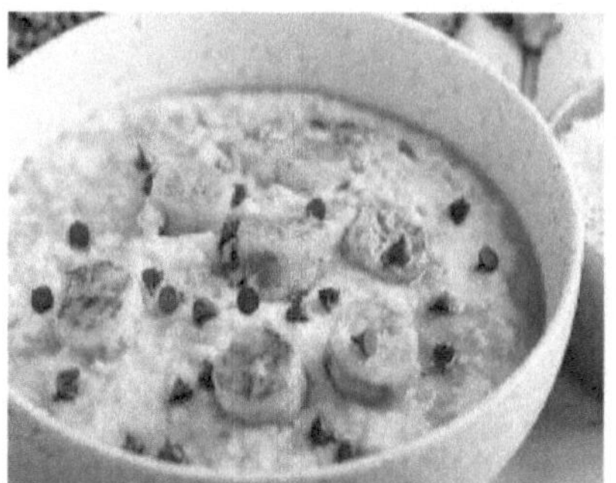

130.　Vitamins Packed Green Juice

Preparation Time: 10 minutes

Cooking Time:0 minutes

Servings: 2

Ingredients:

6 pears, cored and chopped

3 celery stalks

3 C. fresh kale

2 tbsp. fresh parsley

Directions:

Place all the ingredients in a blender and pulse until well combined.

Through a cheesecloth-lined strainer, strain the juice and transfer into 2 glasses.

Serve immediately.

Nutrition:

Calories per serving: 209; Carbohydrates: 50.5g; Protein: 5.1g; Fat: 0.9g; Sugar: 26.2g; Sodium: 66mg; Fiber: 15.2g

131.　Healthier Breakfast Juice

Preparation Time: 10 minutes

Cooking Time:0 minutes

Servings: 2

Ingredients:

2 large Granny Smith apples, cored and sliced

4 medium carrots, peeled and chopped

2 medium grapefruit, peeled and seeded

1 C. fresh kale

1 tsp. fresh lemon juice

Directions:

Place all the ingredients in a blender and pulse until well combined.

Through a cheesecloth-lined strainer, strain the juice and transfer into 2 glasses.

Serve immediately.

Nutrition:

Calories per serving: 265; Carbohydrates: 67g; Protein: 4.2g; Fat: o.7g; Sugar: 47.1g; Sodium: 101mg; Fiber: 11.7g

132.   Summer Perfect Smoothie

Preparation Time: 10 minutes

Servings: 2

Ingredients:

2 C. frozen peaches, pitted

½ C. rolled oats

¼ tsp. ground cinnamon

1½ C. plain yogurt

½ C. fresh orange Juice

Directions:

In a high-speed blender, add all the ingredients and pulse until smooth and creamy.

Transfer the smoothie into 2 serving glasses and serve immediately.

Nutrition:

Calories per serving: 328; Carbohydrates: 56g; Protein: 15g; Fat: 4.1g; Sugar: 41g; Sodium: 131mg; Fiber: 5g

133.   Filling Breakfast Smoothie

Preparation Time: 10 minutes

Cooking Time:0 minutes

Servings: 4

Ingredients:

2 oz. rolled oats

4 apples, peeled, cored and chopped roughly

4 scoops unsweetened vegan protein powder

1 tsp. stevia powder

1 tsp. ground cinnamon

1 tsp. ground nutmeg

17 oz. plain yogurt

2 C. milk

Directions:

In a high-speed blender, add all the ingredients and pulse until smooth and creamy.

Transfer the smoothie into 4 serving glasses and serve immediately.

Nutrition:

Calories per serving: 437; Carbohydrates: 55.6g; Protein: 38.7g; Fat: 6.6g; Sugar: 37.5g; Sodium: 409mg; Fiber: 7.3g

134.   Bright Green Breakfast Bowl

Preparation Time: 10 minutes

Cooking Time:0 minutes

Servings: 2

Ingredients:

2 C. fresh spinach

1 medium avocado, peeled, pitted and chopped roughly

2 scoops unsweetened vegan protein powder

3 tbsp. maple syrup

2 tbsp. fresh lemon juice

1 C. milk

¼ C. ice cubes

Directions:

In a high-speed blender, place all ingredients and pulse until creamy.

Pour into 2 serving bowls and serve immediately with your favorite topping.

Nutrition:

Calories per serving: 471; Carbohydrates: 36.2g; Protein: 32.2g; Fat: 23.5g; Sugar: 24.3g; Sodium: 357mg; Fiber: 8g

135.   Quickest Breakfast Porridge

Cooking Time: 4 minutes

Preparation Time: 10 minutes

Servings: 4

Ingredients:

2 C. milk

3 large apples, peeled, cored and grated

½ tsp. vanilla extract

Pinch of ground cinnamon

1 banana, peeled and sliced

½ small apple, cored and sliced

Directions:

In a large pan, add the milk, grated apples, vanilla extract and cinnamon and mix well.

Place the pan over medium-low heat and cook for about 3-4 minutes, stirring occasionally.

Transfer the porridge into the serving bowls.

Top with the banana and apple slices and serve.

Nutrition:

Calories per serving: 194; Carbohydrates: 40.9g; Protein: 5.9g; Fat: 3g; Sugar: 30g; Sodium: 60mg; Fiber: 6g

136.   Halloween Morning Oatmeal

Preparation Time: 10 minutes

Cooking Time: 2 minutes

Servings: 2

Ingredients:

2 C. hot water

1/3 C. pumpkin puree

1/3 C. rolled oats

1 tsp. ground cinnamon

1 tsp. ground ginger

¼ tsp. ground nutmeg

2 scoops unsweetened vanilla vegan protein powder

1 tbsp. maple syrup

1 small banana, peeled and sliced

Directions:

In a microwave-safe bowl, place water, pumpkin puree, oats, chia seeds and spices and mix well.

Microwave on High for about 2 minutes.

Remove the bowl of oatmeal from the microwave and stir in the protein powder and maple syrup.

Top with banana slices and serve immediately.

Nutrition:

Calories per serving: 268; Carbohydrates: 34.4g; Protein: 28.4g; Fat: 2.4g; Sugar: 14.8g; Sodium: 269mg; Fiber: 5g

137.   Authentic Bulgur Porridge

Preparation Time: 10 minutes

Cooking Time: 15 minutes

Servings: 2

Ingredients:

2/3 C. milk

1/3 C. bulgur, rinsed

Pinch of salt

1 ripe banana, peeled and mashed

1 large apple, peeled, cored and chopped

Directions:

In a pan, add the soy milk, bulgur and salt over medium-high heat and bring to a boil.

Reduce the heat to low and simmer for about 10 minutes.

Remove the pan of bulgur from heat and immediately, stir in the mashed banana.

Serve warm with the topping of chopped apple.

Nutrition:

Calories per serving: 231; Carbohydrates: 50.6g; Protein: 6.5g; Fat: 2.4g;

Sugar: 22.6g; Sodium: 121mg; Fiber: 8.5g

138.   2-Grains Porridge

Preparation Time: 10 minutes

Cooking Time: 20 minutes

Servings: 3

Ingredients:

2 C. milk

2 C. water

1 C. old-fashioned oats

1/3 C. dried quinoa, rinsed

3 tbsp. maple syrup

½ tsp. vanilla extract

1 large banana, peeled and sliced

1 small apple, peeled, cored and chopped

Directions:

In a pan, mix together all the ingredients except for banana and apple over medium heat and bring to a gentle boil.

Cook for about 20 minutes, stirring occasionally.

Remove from the heat and serve warm with the garnishing of banana and apple.

Nutrition:

Calories per serving: 384; Carbohydrates: 72g; Protein: 12.2g; Fat: 6.5g; Sugar: 32.9g; Sodium: 87mg; Fiber: 7g

139.   Savory Crepes

Preparation Time: 10 minutes

Cooking Time: 20 minutes

Servings: 4

Ingredients:

1¼ C. chickpea flour

1½ C. water

¼ tsp. red chili powder

Salt, as required

Directions:

In a blender, add all the ingredients and pulse until well combined.

Heat a lightly greased nonstick skillet over medium-high heat.

Add the desired amount of the mixture and tilt the pan to spread it evenly.

Cook for about 3 minutes.

Carefully, flip the crepe and cook for about 1-2 minutes.

Repeat with the remaining mixture.

Serve warm.

Nutrition:

Calories per serving: 229; Carbohydrates: 38.1g; Protein: 12.1g; Fat: 3.8g; Sugar: 6.7g; Sodium: 55mg; Fiber: 11g

140.   Egg-Free Omelet

Preparation Time: 15 minutes

Cooking Time: 12 minutes

Servings: 4

Ingredients:

1 C. chickpea flour

¼ tsp. ground turmeric

¼ tsp. red chili powder

Pinch of ground cumin

Pinch of sea salt

1½-2 C. water

1 medium onion, chopped finely

2 medium tomatoes, chopped finely

2 tbsp. fresh cilantro, chopped

2 tbsp. olive oil, divided

Directions:

In a large bowl, add the flour, spices, and salt and mix well.

Slowly, add the water and mix until well combined.

Fold in the onion, tomatoes and cilantro.

In a large non-stick frying pan, heat ½ tbsp. of the oil over medium heat.

Add ½ of the tomato mixture and tilt the pan to spread it.

Cook for about 5-7 minutes.

Place the remaining oil over the "omelet" and carefully flip it over.

Cook for about 4-5 minutes or until golden brown.

Repeat with the remaining mixture.

Nutrition:

Calories per serving: 267; Carbohydrates: 35.7g; Protein: 10.6g; Fat: 10.3g; Sugar: 8.3g; Sodium: 86mg; Fiber: 10.2g

141.　Summer Treat Salad

Preparation Time: 15 minutes

Servings: 4

Ingredients:

2 large avocados, peeled, pitted and chopped

1 large apple, peeled, pitted and chopped

1 large peach, peeled, pitted and chopped

1 C. cantaloupe, peeled and chopped

1 shallot, chopped finely

1 seedless cucumber, peeled and chopped

¼ C. fresh lime juice

¼ C. fresh mint, chopped

6 C. lettuce leaves, torn

Directions:

In a large salad bowl, add all the ingredients and toss to coat well.

Set aside for at least 10-20 minutes before serving.

Nutrition:

Calories per serving: 262; Carbohydrates: 28.7g; Protein: 3.7g; Fat: 17.1g; Sugar: 14.9g; Sodium: 20mg; Fiber: 9.5g

142.   Secretly Amazing Salad

Preparation Time: 15 minutes

Cooking Time: 35 minutes

Servings: 6

Ingredients:

For Lentils:

4 C. water

2 C. dried green lentils, rinsed

2 large garlic cloves, halved lengthwise

2 tbsp. olive oil

For Dressing:

1 garlic clove, minced

¼ C. fresh lemon juice

2 tbsp. olive oil

1 tsp. maple syrup

1 tsp. Dijon mustard

Salt and freshly ground black pepper, to taste

For Salad:

1½ (15-oz.) cans chickpeas, rinsed and drained

2 large avocados, peeled, pitted and chopped

2 C. radishes, trimmed and sliced

¼ C. fresh mint leaves, chopped

Directions:

For lentils: in a medium pot, add all ingredients over medium-high heat and bring to a boil.

Reduce the heat to low and simmer for about 25-35 minutes or until the lentils are cooked through and tender.

Drain the lentils and discard the garlic cloves.

For dressing: add all ingredients in a small bowl and beat until well combined.

In a large serving bowl, add lentils, chickpeas, radishes, avocados and mint and mix.

Add the dressing and toss to coat well.

Serve immediately.

Nutrition:

Calories per serving: 561; Carbohydrates: 66.4g; Protein: 24.9g; Fat: 22.2g; Sugar: 3.2g; Sodium: 96mg; Fiber: 29.2g

Lunch

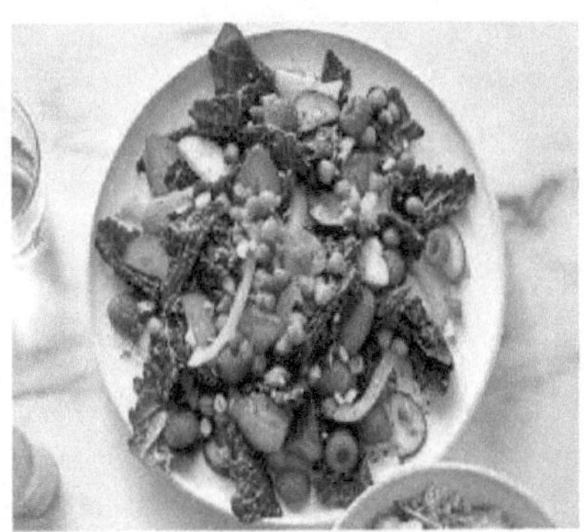

143.   Crowd Pleasing Salad

Preparation Time: 15 minutes

Cooking Time:0 minutes

Servings: 5

Ingredients:

2 C. cooked quinoa

2 C. canned red kidney beans, rinsed and drained

5 C. fresh baby spinach

¼ C. tomatoes, peeled, seeded and chopped

¼ C. fresh dill, chopped

¼ C. fresh parsley, chopped

3 tbsp. fresh lemon juice

Salt and freshly ground black pepper, to taste

Directions:

In a large bowl, add all the ingredients and toss to coat well.

Serve immediately.

Nutrition:

Calories per serving: 354; Carbohydrates: 62.7g; Protein: 16.6g; Fat: 4.8g; Sugar: 2.5g; Sodium: 331mg; Fiber: 11.5g

144.   South Western Salad

Preparation Time: 20 minutes

Cooking Time:0 minutes

Servings: 6

Ingredients:

For Dressing:

2 tbsp. fresh lime juice

2 tbsp. maple syrup

1 tbsp. Dijon mustard

½ tsp. ground cumin

1 tsp. garlic powder

Salt and freshly ground black pepper, to taste

¼ C. extra-virgin olive oil

For Salad:

2 C. fresh mango, peeled, pitted and cubed

2 tbsp. fresh lime juice, divided

2 avocados, peeled, pitted and cubed

Pinch of salt

1 C. cooked quinoa

2 (14-oz.) cans black beans, rinsed and drained

1 small red onion, chopped

½ C. fresh cilantro, chopped

6 C. romaine lettuce, shredded

Directions:

For dressing: in a blender, add all the ingredients except oil and pulse until well combined.

While the motor is running, gradually add the oil and pulse until smooth.

For salad: in a bowl, add the mango and 1 tbsp. of lime juice and toss to coat well.

In another bowl, add the avocado, a pinch of salt and remaining lime juice and toss to coat well.

In a large serving bowl, add the mango, avocado and remaining salad ingredients and mix.

Place the dressing and toss to coat well.

Serve immediately.

Nutrition:

Calories per serving: 555; Carbohydrates: 71.5g; Protein: 18.1g; Fat: 24.4g; Sugar: 13g; Sodium: 69mg; Fiber: 19.7g

145.   Great Luncheon Salad

Preparation Time: 20 minutes

Servings: 4

Ingredients:

For Salad:

½ C. homemade vegetable broth

½ C. couscous

3 C. canned red kidney beans, rinsed and drained

2 large tomatoes, peeled, seeded and chopped

5 C. fresh spinach, torn

For Dressing:

1 garlic clove, minced

2 tbsp. shallots, minced

2 tsp. lemon zest, grated finely

¼ C. fresh lemon juice

2 tbsp. extra-virgin olive oil

Salt and freshly ground black pepper, to taste

Directions:

In a pan, add the broth over medium heat and bring to a boil.

Add the couscous and stir to combine.

Cover the pan and immediately remove from the heat.

Set aside, covered for about 5-10 minutes or until all the liquid is absorbed.

For salad: in a large serving bowl, add the couscous and remaining ingredients and stir to combine.

For dressing: in another small bowl, add all the ingredients and beat until well combined.

Pour the dressing over salad and gently toss to coat well.

Serve immediately.

Nutrition:

Calories per serving: 341; Carbohydrates: 53.2g; Protein: 15.7g; Fat: 8.5g; Sugar: 6.6g; Sodium: 670mg; Fiber: 13.5g

146.   Flavors Powerhouse Lunch Meal

Preparation Time: 15 minutes

Cooking Time: 5 minutes

Servings: 2

Ingredients:

1 large avocado

1¼ C. cooked chickpeas

¼ C. celery stalks, chopped

1 scallion (greed part), sliced

1 small garlic clove, minced

1½ tbsp. fresh lemon juice

½ tsp. olive oil

Salt and freshly ground black pepper, to taste

1 tbsp. fresh cilantro, chopped

Directions:

Cut the avocado in half and then remove the pit.

With a spoon, scoop out the flesh from each avocado half.

Then, cut half of the avocado flesh in equal-sized cubes.

In a large bowl, add avocado cubes and remaining ingredients except for sunflower seeds and cilantro and toss to coat well.

Stuff each avocado half with chickpeas mixture evenly.

Serve immediately with the garnishing of cilantro.

Nutrition:

Calories per serving: 403; Carbohydrates: 0g; Protein: 9.8g; Fat: 22.6g; Sugar: 1.1g; Sodium: 546mg; Fiber: 13.8g

147.   Eye-Catching Sweet Potato Boats

Preparation Time: 20 minutes

Cooking Time: 40 minutes

Servings: 2

Ingredients:

For Sweet Potatoes:

1 large sweet potato, halved lengthwise

½ tbsp. olive oil

Salt and freshly ground black pepper, to taste

For Filling:

½ tbsp. olive oil

1/3 C. canned chickpeas, rinsed and drained

1 tsp. curry powder

1/8 tsp. garlic powder

1/3 C. cooked quinoa

Salt and freshly ground black pepper, to taste

1 tsp. fresh lime juice

1 tsp. fresh cilantro, chopped

Directions:

Preheat the oven to 375 degrees F.

Rub each sweet potato half with oil evenly.

Arrange the sweet potato halves onto a baking sheet, cut side down and sprinkle with salt and black pepper.

Bake for about 40 minutes or until sweet potato becomes tender.

Meanwhile, for filling: in a skillet, heat the oil over medium heat and cook the chickpeas, curry powder and garlic powder for about 6-8 minutes, stirring frequently.

Stir in the cooked quinoa, salt and black pepper and remove from the heat.

Remove from the oven and arrange each sweet potato halves onto a plate.

With a fork, fluff the flesh of each half slightly.

Place chickpeas mixture in each half and drizzle with lime juice

Serve immediately with the garnishing of cilantro and sesame seeds.

Nutrition:

Calories per serving: 286; Carbohydrates: 43g; Protein: 8.2g; Fat: 9.7g; Sugar: 6.6g; Sodium: 175mg; Fiber: 8g

148.   Mexican Enchiladas

Preparation Time: 15 minutes

Cooking Time: 20 minutes

Servings: 8

Ingredients:

1 (14-oz.) can red beans, drained, rinsed and mashed

2 C. cheddar cheese, grated

2 C. tomato sauce

½ C. onion, chopped

¼ C. black olives, pitted and sliced

2 tsp. garlic salt

8 whole-wheat tortillas

Directions:

Preheat the oven to 350 degrees F.

In a medium bowl, add the mashed beans, cheese, 1 C. of tomato sauce, onions, olives and garlic salt and mix well.

Place about 1/3 C. of the bean mixture along center of each tortilla.

Roll up each tortilla and place enchiladas in large baking dish.

Place the remaining tomato sauce on top of the filled tortillas.

Bake for about 15-20 minutes.

Serve warm.

Nutrition:

Calories per serving: 358; Carbohydrates: 46.2g; Protein: 20.6g; Fat: 11.2g; Sugar: 4.5g; Sodium: 550mg; Fiber: 10.3g

149. Unique Banana Curry

Preparation Time: 15 minutes

Cooking Time: 15 minutes

Servings: 3

Ingredients:

2 tbsp. olive oil

2 yellow onions, chopped

8 garlic cloves, minced

2 tbsp. curry powder

1 tbsp. ground ginger

1 tbsp. ground cumin

1 tsp. ground turmeric

1 tsp. ground cinnamon

1 tsp. red chili powder

Salt and freshly ground black pepper, to taste

2/3 C. plain yogurt

1 C. tomato puree

2 bananas, peeled and sliced

3 tomatoes, peeled, seeded and chopped finely

Directions:

In a large pan, heat the oil over medium heat and sauté onion for about 4-5 minutes.

Add the garlic, curry powder and spices and sauté for about 1 minute.

Add the yogurt and tomato sauce and bring to a gentle boil.

Stir in the bananas and simmer for about 3 minutes.

Stir in the tomatoes and simmer for about 1-2 minutes.

Remove from the heat and serve hot.

Nutrition:

Calories per serving: 318; Carbohydrates: 49.7g; Protein: 9g; Fat: 12.2g; Sugar: 24.2g; Sodium: 138mg; Fiber: 9.5g

150.   Vegan-Friendly Platter

Preparation Time: 10 minutes

Cooking Time: 30 minutes

Servings: 4

Ingredients:

1 tbsp. olive oil

2 small onions, chopped

5 garlic cloves, chopped finely

1 tsp. of dried oregano

1 tsp. ground cumin

½ tsp. ground ginger

Salt and freshly ground black pepper, to taste

2 cups tomatoes, peeled, seeded and chopped

2 (13½-oz.) cans black beans, rinsed and drained

½ C. homemade vegetable broth

Directions:

In a pan, heat the olive oil over medium heat and cook the onion for about 5-7 minutes, stirring frequently.

Add the garlic, oregano, spices, salt and black pepper and cook for about 1 minute.

Add the tomatoes and cook for about 1-2 minutes.

Add in the beans and broth and bring to a boil.

Reduce the heat to medium-low and simmer, covered for about 15 minutes.

Serve hot.

Nutrition:

Calories per serving: 327; Carbohydrates: 54.1g; Protein: 19.1g; Fat: 5.1g; Sugar: 4g; Sodium: 595mg; Fiber: 18.8g

151.   Armenian Style Chickpeas

Preparation Time: 15 minutes

Cooking Time: 15 minutes

Servings: 4

Ingredients:

2 tbsp. olive oil

1 medium yellow onion, chopped

4 garlic cloves, minced

1 tsp. dried thyme, crushed

1 tsp. dried oregano, crushed

½ tsp. paprika

1 C. tomato, chopped finely

2½ C. canned chickpeas, rinsed and drained

5 C. Swiss chard, chopped

2 tbsp. water

2 tbsp. fresh lemon juice

Salt and freshly ground black pepper, to taste

3 tbsp. fresh basil, chopped

Directions:

In a skillet, heat the olive oil over medium heat and sauté the onion for about 6-8 minutes.

Add the garlic, herbs and paprika and sauté for about 1 minute.

Add the Swiss chard and 2 tbsp. water and cook for about 2-3 minutes.

Add the tomatoes and chickpeas and cook for about 2-3 minutes.

Add in the lemon juice, salt and black pepper and remove from the heat.

Serve hot with the garnishing of basil.

Nutrition:

Calories per serving: 260; Carbohydrates: 34g; Protein: 12g; Fat: 8.6g; Sugar: 3.1g; Sodium: 178mg; Fiber: 9g

152. Protein-Packed Soup

Preparation Time: 15 minutes

Cooking Time: 1 hour 10 minutes

Servings: 8

Ingredients:

2 tbsp. olive oil

1½ lb. ground turkey

Salt and freshly ground black pepper, to taste

1 large carrot, peeled and chopped

1 large celery stalk, chopped

1 large onion, chopped

6 garlic cloves, chopped

1 tsp. dried rosemary

1 tsp. dried oregano

2 large potatoes, peeled and chopped

8-9 C. chicken bone broth

4-5 C. tomatoes, peeled, seeded and chopped

2 C. dry lentils

¼ C. fresh parsley, chopped

Directions:

In a large soup pan, heat the olive oil over medium-high heat and cook the turkey for about 5 minutes or until browned.

With a slotted spoon, transfer the turkey into a bowl and set aside.

In the same pan, add the carrot, celery onion, garlic and dried herbs over medium heat and cook for about 5 minutes.

Add the potatoes and cook for about 4-5 minutes.

Add the cooked turkey, tomatoes and broth and bring to a boil over high heat.

Reduce the heat to low and cook, covered for about 10 minutes.

Add the lentils and cook, covered for about 40 minutes.

Stir in black pepper and remove from the heat.

Serve hot with the garnishing of parsley.

Nutrition:

Calories per serving: 485; Carbohydrates: 44.6g; Protein: 43g; Fat: 16.5g; Sugar: 8.5g; Sodium: 452mg; Fiber: 16.6g

153.   One-Pot Dinner Soup

Preparation Time: 15 minutes

Cooking Time: 50 minutes

Servings: 4

Ingredients:

1 tbsp. olive oil

1 C. yellow onion, chopped

½ C. carrots, peeled and chopped

½ C. celery, chopped

2 garlic cloves, minced

4 C. homemade vegetable broth

2½ C. sweet potatoes, peeled and chopped

1 C. red lentils, rinsed

1½ tbsp. fresh lemon juice

Salt and freshly ground black pepper, to taste

2 tbsp. fresh cilantro, chopped

Directions:

In a large Dutch oven, heat the oil over medium heat and sauté the onion, carrot and celery for about 5-7 minutes.

Add the garlic and sauté for about 1 minute.

Add the sweet potatoes and cook for about 1-2 minutes.

Add in the broth and bring to a boil.

Reduce the heat to low and simmer, covered for about 5 minutes.

Stir in the red lentils and gain bring to a boil over medium-high heat.

Reduce the heat to low and simmer, covered for about 25-30 minutes or until desired doneness.

Stir in the lemon juice, salt and black pepper and remove from the heat.

Serve hot with the garnishing of cilantro.

Nutrition:

Calories per serving: 471; Carbohydrates: 61g; Protein: 19,3g; Fat: 5.6g; Sugar: 4.4g; Sodium: 836mg; Fiber: 19.7g

154.   3-Beans Soup

Preparation Time: 15 minutes

Cooking Time: 45 minutes

Ingredients:

¼ C. olive oil

1 large onion, chopped

1 large sweet potato, peeled and cubed

3 carrots, peeled and chopped

3 celery stalks, chopped

3 garlic cloves, minced

2 tsp. dried thyme, crushed

1 tbsp. red chili powder

1 tbsp. ground cumin

4 large tomatoes, peeled, seeded and chopped finely

2 (16-oz.) cans great Northern beans, rinsed and drained

2 (15¼-oz.) cans red kidney beans, rinsed and drained

1 (15-oz.) can black beans, drained and rinsed

12 C. homemade vegetable broth

1 C. fresh cilantro, chopped

Salt and freshly ground black pepper, to taste

Directions:

In a Dutch oven, heat the oil over medium heat and sauté the onion, sweet potato, carrot and celery for about 6-8 minutes.

Add the garlic, thyme, chili powder and cumin and sauté for about 1 minute.

Add in the tomatoes and cook for about 2-3 minutes.

Add the beans and broth and bring to a boil over medium-high heat.

Cover the pan with lid and cook for about 25-30 minutes.

Stir in the cilantro and remove from heat.

Serve hot.

Nutrition:

Calories per serving: 411; Carbohydrates: 69.7g; Protein: 22.7g; Fat: 5.7g; Sugar: 7.1g; Sodium: 931mg; Fiber: 18.9g

## 155.	Pork and Penne Pasta

Preparation Time: 20 mins.

Cooking Time: 30 mins.

Servings: 4

Ingredients:

whole wheat penne pasta (1 lb.)

ground Pork lean (1 lb)

extra virgin olive oil (2 tbs)

onion (1 small, chopped)

garlic cloves (2, minced)

can tomatoes (1 (15 oz), diced, seeded)

green zucchini (2 cups sliced to 1/4 cubes)

baby spinach (8 oz., fresh, chopped)

low fat parmesan cheese (1 cup, grated)

Directions:

Bring a pot of water to a boil, ensure that the water is salted. Cook the pasta to an al dente consistency or according to package directions.

In a non-stick pan, cook the ground Pork over medium heat for 8 minutes or until it is browned, ensure to break up any large pieces in the pan.

Remove Pork and set aside. Discard drippings. Add in your oil on medium heat.

Cook onions and garlic for about 5 minutes or until soft. Add tomatoes and zucchini and continue cooking 5 minutes more.

Add spinach and cook until it just wilts, 2-3 minutes. Place the Pork back into the skillet and add 1/2 cup cheese; stir and heat through.

Plate your pasta then top with your meat mixture. Toss well and top evenly with cheese.

Nutrition:

206 calories, 9 g fat, 24g carbs, 13 g fiber, 17 g protein

156. Chicken and Quinoa Pita

Preparation Time: 10 mins.

Cooking Time: 0 mins.

Servings: 4

Ingredients:

fat free cream cheese (1 cup, softened)

fat free mayonnaise (1 tbs)

cooked chicken (2 cups, cubed)

tomatoes (1 cup, seeded, sliced)

Quinoa (1 (14 oz) can, cooked)

romaine lettuce leaves (4)

alfalfa sprouts (2 cups, rinsed, drained)

whole wheat pita bread (4 round)

Directions:

In a bowl, combine mayonnaise and cream cheese until it is fully mixed. Add chicken, tomatoes, Quinoa; mix well. Slice the pita bread to form a pocket. Fill your pitas with lettuce and chicken. Top with alfalfa sprouts. Serve.

Nutrition:

331 calories, 23 g fat, 5 g carbs, 2 g fiber, 26 g protein

157. Chicken and Asparagus Pasta

Preparation Time: 10 mins.

Cooking Time: 22 mins.

Servings: 4

Ingredients:

whole wheat penne pasta (1 lb.)

olive oil (2 tbs)

chicken breast halves (3/4 lb, sliced into strips)

poultry seasoning (1/2 tsp)

cloves garlic (4, minced)

asparagus (1 1/2 cup, frozen, cut into 1 inch)

peas (1 cup, frozen, thawed)

parmesan cheese (1/4 cup, grated)

Directions:

Bring a pot of salted water to boil. Add pasta and cook to an al dente consistency according to package directions.

Heat one tablespoon olive oil in a non-stick pan over medium heat and cook chicken with poultry seasoning until golden.

Remove cooked chicken from the pan.

Add the remaining tablespoon of olive oil, garlic, asparagus and peas. Cook until vegetables are tender.

Put the chicken back into the pan with the asparagus mixture and cook for 2 minutes.

Put the pasta in a shallow pasta bowl and toss with chicken mixture. Top with parmesan cheese.

Nutrition:

168 calories, 10 g fat, 7g carbs, 3 g fiber, 13 g protein

158.   Turkey Florentine

Preparation Time: 15 mins.

Cooking Time: 18 mins.

Servings: 4

Ingredients:

olive oil (2 tbs)

zucchinis (2 medium, seeded, thinly sliced)

green onions (1/2 cups, sliced)

turkey breast (2 cups, cubed)

salt (1/2 tsp)

thyme (1/2 tsp, ground)

pimento (2 tbs, chopped)

cooked long-grain rice (3 cups)

fresh baby spinach (4 cups)

low fat parmesan cheese (1/4 cup, freshly grated)

Directions:

In a non-stick pan, heat olive oil over moderate heat. Add zucchini, turkey, and onions, stir ever now and then for 5 to 10 minutes.

Add salt, thyme, pimento, rice and spinach. Cook and stir for another 6 - 8 minutes or until heated through and spinach wilts.

Remove from heat, transfer to large serving bowl, and stir in cheese. Serve.

Nutrition:

593 calories, 8 g fat, 11 g carbs, 4 g fiber, 12 g protein

159.   Chicken Lettuce Wraps

Preparation Time: 15 mins.

Cooking Time: 0 mins.

Servings: 2

Ingredients:

Mayonnaise (1/4 cup, low fat)

lemon juice (2 tsp)

white beans (1/2 cup, canned, cooked, drained)

feta cheese (1/3 cup, crumbled)

pimentos (2 tbs, chopped)

lettuce leaves (8 large, washed, and dried)

chicken breast strips (1/2 lb cooked, preferably grilled)

Directions:

In a medium bowl, combine mayonnaise and lemon juice. Stir in beans, mashing slightly with fork. Add cheese and pimentos and mix lightly. Spread lettuce leaves evenly with bean mixture. Top with chicken; roll up. Serve.

Nutrition:

338 calories, 10 g fat, 39g carbs, 9 g fiber, 26 g protein

160.   Couscous with Turkey

Preparation Time: 20 mins.

Cooking Time: 26 mins.

Servings: 4

Ingredients:

extra-virgin olive oil (4 tbs)

turkey thighs (1 lb boneless, skinless, chopped)

onion (1, chopped)

cloves garlic (3, minced)

carrots (1 cup, shredded)

smoked paprika (1 tsp)

ground cinnamon (1/8 tsp)

salt (1/2 tsp)

dried fruits (1 cup chopped, pitted dates, apricots)

turkey stock (4 cups, divided)

butter (2 tablespoons)

couscous (1 1/2 cups)

Italian parsley (1/2 cup, chopped)

Directions:

Set your oil to get hot on medium heat. Cook turkey and brown 3 to 4 minutes on each side.

Add onions, garlic, carrots, and season with spices and salt. Cook 6-8 minutes.

Stir the fruits into the turkey and vegetables, and 2 ½ cups of stock.

Allow to boil. Turn down the heat to low, cover and let it simmer for 10 minutes.

In a separate small saucepan, over medium heat, pour 1 ½ cups of stock and bring up to a boil then stir in the couscous.

Take the content off the heat and let it stand 5 minutes while the cover is on. Fluff with fork and serve with turkey.

Nutrition:

469 calories, 24 g fat, 40 g carbs, 4 g fiber, 18 g protein

161.   <u>Easy Turkey Chili</u>

Preparation Time: 25 mins.

Cooking Time: 47 mins.

Servings: 4-6

Ingredients:

olive oil (3 tbs)

garlic cloves (4, minced)

onion (1 medium, chopped)

ground turkey (1 lb.)

bay leaf (1)

ground cumin (1 tsp)

dried oregano (1 tsp)

tomato (1, seeded and chopped)

tomato sauce (1 (14 oz.) can)

Pork broth (1 cup

salt (1 tsp)

red beans (2 (14 oz.) cans, drained and rinsed)

Directions:

Heat the oil over medium heat, in a large pot and cook the onions and garlic for 5 minutes.

Turn the heat from medium to high. Add oregano, bay leaf, turkey and cumin. Cook for 5-7 minutes or until turkey has browned.

Add broth, tomato sauce, tomato and salt. Once the pot is boiling, lower the heat to simmer. Let it simmer for about 20 minutes, covered.

If needed, add more water and beans and continue to simmer for 15 more minutes. Serve.

Nutrition:

193 calories, 13 g fat, 5 g carbs, 1 g fiber, 16 g protein

162.   Ham, Bean and Cabbage Stew

Preparation Time: 15 mins.

Cooking Time: 17 mins.

Servings: 4

Ingredients:

extra virgin olive oil (1 tbs)

smoked ham (8 oz, chopped)

onion (1 large, chopped)

stalks celery (2, sliced)

cloves garlic (5, chopped finely)

chicken broth (4 cups)

tomatoes (1 (28 oz) can, seedless, drained)

whole wheat pasta (3 cups)

coleslaw (8 oz)

kidney beans (2 (14 oz) cans)

dried basil (1 tsp)

dried rosemary (1 tsp)

Directions:

In a good size pot, heat olive oil over medium heat. Cook ham, onion, celery and garlic stirring occasionally, until vegetables are tender.

Stir in broth and tomatoes, breaking up tomatoes. Stir the pasta in, heat to boiling and turn down the heat low.

Cover and simmer about 10 minutes or until pasta is tender. Stir in coleslaw, beans, basil and oregano.

Bring stew to a boil and reduce heat to low. Simmer uncovered about 5-7 minutes or until cabbage is tender.

Nutrition:

543 calories, 21 g fat, 47g carbs, 8 g fiber, 40 g protein

163.   Grilled Fish Tacos

Preparation Time: 25 mins.

Cooking Time: 6 mins.

Servings: 4

Ingredients:

Salt (1/4 tsp)

Juice of 1/2 lemon

olive oil (2 tbs)

trout filets (4, rinsed and dried)

red onion (1/2 cup, chopped)

jicama (1/2 cup, peeled, chopped)

red bell pepper (1/3 cup, chopped)

fresh cilantro (2/3 cup, finely chopped)

black beans (1 cup, drained and rinsed)

Zest and juice (1/2 lime)

plain yogurt (1 tbs, non-fat)

whole wheat tortillas (8, warmed)

Directions:

Combine your oil, lemon juice and salt.

Pour mixture over fish fillets and let marinate for 10 minutes. Put the fish on the grill over high heat.

Cook the fish on both side for 3 minutes. In another bowl, combine onion, bell pepper, jicama, cilantro, yogurt and zest and juice of lime to make a salsa.

Add your fish on top of a warm tortilla. Top with salsa and fold in half before serving.

Nutrition:

356 calories, 9 g fat, 57g carbs, 17 g fiber, 15 g protein

164.   Pasta with Turkey and Olives

Preparation Time: 20 mins.

Cooking Time: 30 mins.

Servings: 4

Ingredients:

whole wheat pasta (1 lb, uncooked)

olive oil (2 tsp)

onion (1 large, peeled, chopped finely)

cloves garlic (4, peeled, finely chopped)

turkey breast (1 lb, cut into chunks)

basil (1 tsp, dried)

rosemary (1 tsp, dried)

black olives (12 med, pitted)

green bell pepper (1 med, seeded and chopped)

tomatoes (1 (14 oz) can, seedless, chopped)

chicken broth (1 can)

Romano cheese (1/2 cup, shredded)

Directions:

Bring a salted water to boil in a large pot. Add pasta and cook until al dente follow instruction according to the package.

While pasta cooks, heat the oil in a large pan over medium heat. Add the garlic and onion. Cook for 6 minutes.

Add the turkey, rosemary and basil. Cook for about 8 minutes.

Stir in the olives, tomatoes and green pepper and cook for 2 minutes. In the pan add the chicken broth, heat the pan to a boil.

Reduce half of the liquid by boiling for 7 minutes. When pasta is done, add to sauce mixture.

Toss until pasta is evenly mixed with sauce. Top with cheese and serve.

Nutrition:

165 calories, 4 g fat, 18 g carbs, 3 g fiber, 14 g protein

Snack

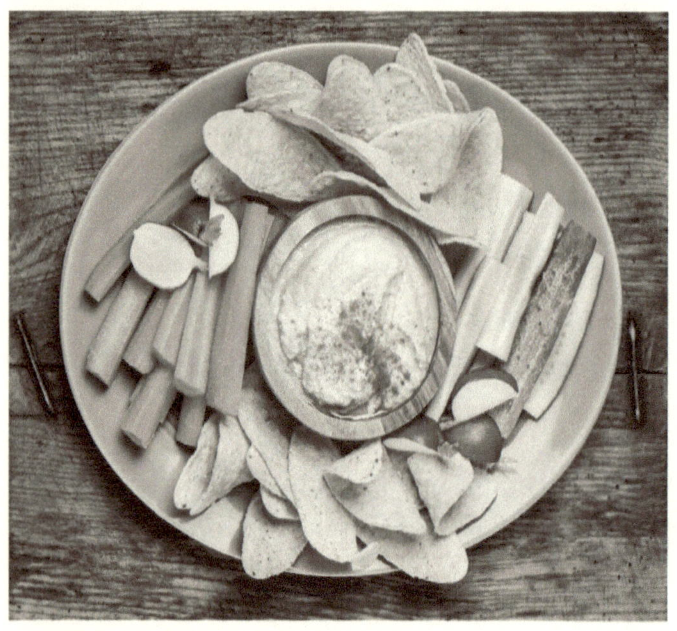

165.   Ricotta & Cannellini Salad

Preparation Time: 15 mins.

Cooking Time: 0 mins.

Servings: 6

Ingredients:

plain yogurt (2 tbs, low fat)

extra virgin olive oil (3 tbs)

fresh lemon juice (2 tbs)

oregano (3/4 tsp, ground)

fresh mint (1 tbs, shredded)

white cannellini beans (2 (14 oz) cans, drained and rinsed)

red onions (1/2 cup, thinly sliced)

tomatoes (3 medium, seeded and chopped)

Greek olives (1/4 cup, pitted)

ricotta cheese (1/2 cup, crumbled)

spinach leaves (2 cups)

Directions:

In large bowl, combine yogurt, olive oil, lemon juice, oregano, and mint; whisk well.

Add onion, beans, tomato, ricotta cheese and olives; toss lightly.

Refrigerate for at least one hour. Serve on a bed of spinach.

Nutrition:

160 calories, 11 g fat, 10 g carbs, 2 g fiber, 6 g protein

166.   Bean and Tomato Salad

Preparation Time: 10 mins.

Cooking Time: 0 mins.

Servings: 4

Ingredients:

Tomatoes (4 medium, seeded and chopped)

garbanzos (2 (14 oz) cans, drained and rinsed)

red onions (1/4 cup, chopped finely)

Italian parsley (1 cup, chopped finely)

lemon Juice (2 tbs)

extra virgin olive oil (1/4 cup)

salt (1/2 tsp)

Directions:

Combine your parsley, onions, beans and tomato. Set aside. In another bowl whisk together salt, olive oil and lemon juice.

Pour dressing over vegetables. Mix and serve.

Nutrition:

201 calories, 14 g fat, 18 g carbs, 4 g fiber, 4 g protein

## 167.	String bean Potato Salad

Preparation Time: 15 mins.

Cooking Time: 7 mins.

Servings: 4-6

Ingredients:

string beans (1 1/2 lbs, slender)

red potatoes (6 small, unpeeled, cubed)

red onion (1 small, thinly sliced lengthwise)

extra virgin olive oil (1/3 cup)

red wine vinegar (1/4 cup)

rice vinegar (1/4 cup)

garlic salt (1 tbs)

sugar (1 tsp)

Directions:

In a pot of boiling water, cook potatoes and string beans about 7 minutes.

Drain the contents and run cold water on the beans only to stop cooking process. Drain and set it aside.

In a large salad bowl, combine beans, potatoes and onions. For dressing, in a bowl, whisk together olive oil, vinegars, garlic salt and sugar.

Toss the vegetables and dressing together until coated. Refrigerate one hour prior to serving.

Nutrition:

142 calories, 11 g fat, 10g carbs, 1 g fiber, 1 g protein

168.   Cucumber Peach Salad

Preparation Time: 30 mins.

Cooking Time: 0 mins.

Servings: 4

Ingredients:

Avocados (2 large, pitted and diced)

Peach (1, unpeeled, pitted and diced)

Gala pear (1, unpeeled, cored and diced)

Cantaloupe (1 cup, chopped)

Shallot (1, chopped finely)

English cucumber (1, chopped)

fresh lime juice (1/4 cup)

fresh mint (1/4 cup, chopped)

Large lettuce leaves

Directions:

In a medium bowl, combine all ingredients except the lettuce leaves. Sprinkle the mint and lime juice.

Toss until combine. Let salad sit at least 10-20 minutes. Serve over 2 leaves of lettuce per serving.

Nutrition:

182 calories, 11 g fat, 23g carbs, 3 g fiber, 6 g protein

169.   Strawberry & Apple Salad

Preparation Time: 10 mins.

Cooking Time: 0 mins.

Servings: 2

Ingredients:

Ripe strawberries (1½ cups)

Fresh apple (cut in small cubes, 1½ cups)

Brazil nuts (12, blanched and thinly sliced)

Lemon juice (4 tablespoonfuls)

Lettuce

Dressing, (1 tablespoonful)

Directions:

Cut the apples and strawberries and add Brazil nuts that have been marinated in lemon juice.

Shape your lettuce into a rose, and fill the lettuce with the mixture above, and cover with a spoonful salad dressing.

Nutrition:

184 calories, 11 g fat, 23 g carbs, 4 g fiber, 4 g protein

170.   Bean and Couscous Salad

Preparation Time: 15 mins.

Cooking Time: 0 mins.

Servings: 4

Ingredients:

couscous (1 cup)

boiling water (1 1/2 cups)

sweet yellow peppers (1 cup, seeded and chopped)

black beans (2 cups, cooked)

onion (1 small, chopped)

tomatoes (2 cups, seeded and chopped)

garlic cloves (2 medium, minced)

rice vinegar (1/2 cup)

olive oil (1/4 cup)

salt (1/2 tsp)

Directions:

In a large bowl, place the couscous with boiling water. Cover and wait until couscous have absorbed all the water.

Place couscous in a bowl and add the remaining ingredients. Mix well. Serve.

Nutrition:

637 calories, 15 g fat, 101 g carbs, 18 g fiber, 28 g protein

171. Asian Chicken Salad

Preparation Time: 15 mins.

Cooking Time: 0 mins.

Servings: 1

Ingredients:

romaine lettuce (1 cup, chopped)

carrot (1, shredded)

celery (1, sliced thinly)

red pepper (1/4 cup, seeded, sliced thinly)

chicken breast (1/2 cup, cooked, cut into strips)

mangos (1/4 cup, chopped)

lime and ginger dressing (2 tbsp)

Directions:

Toss together all ingredients in a medium bowl until combined. Serve alone or with whole wheat bread slices.

Nutrition:

384 calories, 4 g fat, 68g carbs, 10 g fiber, 25 g protein

172.   Almond Salad

Preparation Time: 10 mins.

Cooking Time: 0 mins.

Servings: 1

Ingredients:

Blanched almonds (1½ cups, chopped)

Olives (18)

Celery (1½ cups, cut fine)

Salad dressing (1 tbs)

Lettuce

Directions:

Stone and chop the olives. Add the almonds and the celery. Mix with salad dressing and serve on the lettuce.

Nutrition:

101 calories, 6 g fat, 10g carbs, 3 g fiber, 2 g protein

173.   Vegetarian Nuttolene Salad

Preparation Time: 10 mins.

Cooking Time: 0 mins.

Servings: 1

Ingredients:

Nuttolene (¼ pound, Chopped)

Celery (2/3 cup, Chopped)

Protose (½ pound, Chopped)

Onion (1 small teaspoonful, Grated)

Lemons juice (2)

Salt.

Mayonnaise (2 tablespoonfuls)

Directions:

Mix all the ingredients together, then add the mayonnaise dressing last. Serve

Nutrition:

55 calories, 0 g fat, 12 g carbs, 3 g fiber, 2 g protein

174.   Nutty Green Salad

Preparation Time: 5 mins.

Cooking Time: 0 mins.

Servings: 4

Ingredients:

Walnut meats (1 cup)

French peas (1 can)

Mayonnaise (1 tbs)

Lettuce (1 medium)

Directions:

Put the walnut meats in extreme hot water for fifteen minutes.

Remove the skins, then cut it into pieces. Set your peas to scald then set aside.

Drain the water from the peas, and let it get cold; then mix with the walnuts.

Add the mayonnaise dressing and mix thoroughly. Serve on lettuce.

Nutrition:

252 calories, 2 g fat, 11 g carbs, 4 g fiber, 10 g protein

Dinner

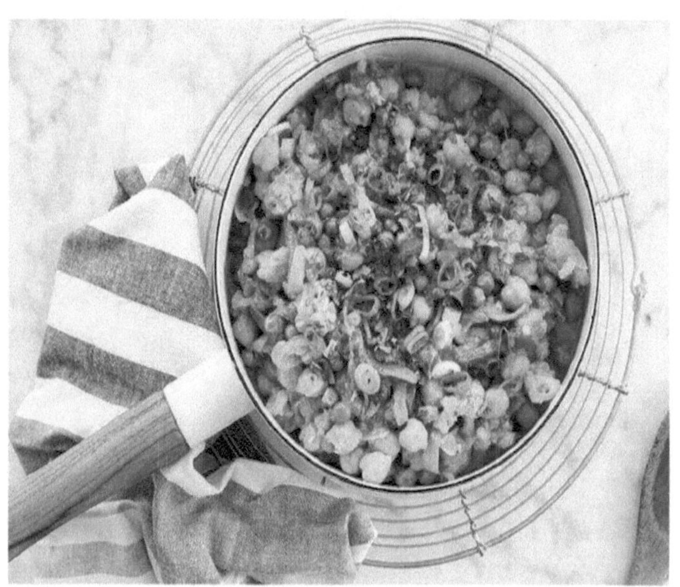

175.   Heavenly Tasty Stew

Preparation Time: 15 minutes

Cooking Time: 35 minutes

Servings: 6

Ingredients:

¼ C. olive oil

1 large yellow onion, chopped

8 oz. fresh shiitake mushrooms, sliced

2 large tomatoes, chopped

2 tbsp. garlic, chopped finely

2 bay leaves

2 tbsp. mixed Italian herbs (rosemary, thyme, basil), chopped

1 tsp. cayenne pepper

4 C. homemade vegetable broth

2 tbsp. apple cider vinegar

1 C. whole-wheat fusilli pasta

1/3 C. nutritional yeast

8 oz. fresh collard greens

1 (15-oz.) can cannellini beans, drained and rinsed

Salt and freshly ground black pepper, to taste

Directions:

In a large pan, heat the oil over medium heat and sauté the onion, mushrooms, potato and tomato for about 4-5 minutes.

Add the garlic, bay leaves, herbs and cayenne pepper and sauté for about 1 minute.

Add the broth and bring to a boil.

Stir in the vinegar, pasta and nutritional yeast and again bring to a boil.

Reduce the heat to medium-low and simmer, covered for about 20 minutes.

Uncover and stir in the greens and beans.

Simmer for about 4-5 minutes.

Stir in the salt and black pepper and remove from the heat.

Serve hot.

Nutrition:

Calories per serving: 314; Carbohydrates: 46g; Protein: 14.4g; Fat: 10g; Sugar: 6.2g; Sodium: 489mg; Fiber: 12.3g

176. Thanksgiving Dinner Chili

Preparation Time: 15 minutes

Cooking Time: 45 minutes

Servings: 6

Ingredients:

2 tbsp. olive oil

1 red bell pepper, seeded and chopped

1 onion, chopped

2 garlic cloves, chopped

1 lb. lean ground turkey

2 C. water

3 C. tomatoes, chopped finely

1 tsp. ground cumin

½ tsp. ground cinnamon

1 (15-oz.) can red kidney beans, rinsed and drained

1 (15-oz.) cans black beans, rinsed and drained

¼ C. scallion greens, chopped

Directions:

In a large Dutch oven, heat the olive oil over medium-low heat and sauté bell pepper, onion and garlic for about 5 minutes.

Add the turkey and cook for about 5-6 minutes, breaking up the chunks with a wooden spoon.

Add the water, tomatoes and spices and bring to a boil over high heat.

Reduce the heat to medium-low and stir in beans and corn.

Simmer, covered for about 30 minutes, stirring occasionally.

Serve hot with the topping of scallion greens.

Nutrition:

Calories per serving: 366; Carbohydrates: 40.6g; Protein: 28.7g; Fat: 11.2g; Sugar: 4.5g; Sodium: 100mg; Fiber: 13.4g

177.   Meatless Monday Chili

Preparation Time: 15 minutes

Cooking Time: 1 hour 25 minutes

Servings: 4

Ingredients:

2 tbsp. avocado oil

1 medium onion, chopped

1 carrot, peeled and chopped

1 small bell pepper, seeded and chopped

1 lb. fresh mushrooms, sliced

2 garlic cloves, minced

2 tsp. dried oregano

1 tbsp. red chili powder

1 tbsp. ground cumin

Salt and freshly ground black pepper, to taste

8 oz. canned red kidney beans, rinsed and drained

8 oz. canned white kidney beans, rinsed and drained

2 C. tomatoes, peeled, seeded and chopped finely

1½ C. homemade vegetable broth

Directions:

In a large Dutch oven, heat the oil over medium-low heat and cook the onions, carrot and bell pepper for about 10 minutes, stirring frequently.

Increase the heat to medium-high.

Stir in the mushrooms and garlic and cook for about 5-6 minutes, stirring frequently.

Add the oregano, spices, salt and black pepper and cook for about chili 1-2 minutes.

Stir in the beans, tomatoes and broth and bring to a boil.

Reduce the heat to low and simmer, covered for about 1 hour, stirring occasionally.

Serve hot.

Nutrition:

Calories per serving: 346; Carbohydrates: 59.9g; Protein: 23.4g; Fat:3.7g; Sugar: 10.5g; Sodium: 545mg; Fiber: 16.7g

178.   Beans Trio Chili

Preparation Time: 15 minutes

Cooking Time: 1 hour

Servings: 6

Ingredients:

2 tbsp. olive oil

1 green bell pepper, seeded and chopped

2 celery stalks, chopped

1 scallion, chopped

3 garlic cloves, minced

1 tsp. dried oregano, crushed

1 tbsp. red chili powder

2 tsp. ground cumin

1 tsp. red pepper flakes, crushed

1 tsp. ground turmeric

1 tsp. onion powder

1 tsp. garlic powder

Salt and freshly ground black pepper, to taste

4½ C. tomatoes, peeled, seeded and chopped finely

4 C. water

1 (16-oz.) can red kidney beans, rinsed and drained

1 (16-oz.) can cannellini beans, rinsed and drained

½ of (16-oz.) can black beans, rinsed and drained

Directions:

In a large pan, heat the oil over medium heat and cook the bell peppers, celery, scallion and garlic for about 8-10 minutes, stirring frequently.

Add the oregano, spices, salt, black pepper, tomatoes and water and bring to a boil.

Simmer for about 20 minutes.

Stir in the beans and simmer for about 30 minutes.

Serve hot.

Nutrition:

Calories per serving: 342; Carbohydrates: 56g; Protein: 20.3g; Fat: 6.1g; Sugar: 6g; Sodium: 79mg; Fiber: 21.3g

179.   Staple Vegan Curry

Preparation Time: 15 minutes

Cooking Time: 40 minutes

Servings: 6

Ingredients:

10 oz. whole-wheat pasta

1 tbsp. vegetable oil

1 medium white onion, chopped

3 garlic cloves, minced

1 tsp. dried basil, crushed

1 tbsp. curry powder

¼ tsp. red pepper flakes, crushed

2 lb. ripe tomatoes, peeled, seeded and chopped

4 C. cauliflower, cut into bite-sized pieces

1 medium red bell pepper, seeded and sliced thinly

1 C. water

1 (15-oz.) can chickpeas, drained and rinsed

1 C. fresh baby spinach

¼ C. fresh parsley, chopped

Salt, to taste

Directions:

In a pan of the salted boiling water, add the pasta and cook for about 8-10 minutes or according to package's directions.

Drain the pasta well and set aside.

Heat the oil in a large cast-iron skillet over medium heat and sauté the onion for about 4-5 minutes.

Add the garlic, basil, curry powder and red pepper flakes and sauté for about 1 minute.

Stir in the tomatoes, cauliflower, bell pepper and water and bring to a gentle boil.

Reduce the heat to medium-low and simmer, covered for about 15-20 minutes.

Stir in the chickpeas and cook for about 5 minutes.

Add the spinach and cook for about 3-4 minutes.

Stir in the pasta and remove from the heat.

Serve hot.

Nutrition:

Calories per serving: 338; Carbohydrates: 58.4g; Protein: 15.1g; Fat: 5.9g; Sugar: 10.9g; Sodium: 80mg; Fiber: 10.3g

180.   Fragrant Vegetarian Curry

Preparation Time: 15 minutes

Cooking Time: 1½ hours

Servings: 8

Ingredients:

8 C. water

½ tsp. ground turmeric

1 C. brown lentils

1 C. red lentils

1 tbsp. olive oil

1 large white onion, chopped

3 garlic cloves, minced

2 large tomatoes, peeled, seeded and chopped

1½ tbsp. curry powder

¼ tsp. ground cloves

2 tsp. ground cumin

3 carrots, peeled and chopped

3 C. pumpkin, peeled, seeded and cubed into 1-inch size

1 granny smith apple, cored and chopped

2 C. fresh spinach, chopped

Salt and freshly ground black pepper, to taste

Directions:

In a large pan, add the water, turmeric and lentils over high heat and bring to a boil.

Reduce the heat to medium-low and simmer, covered for about 30 minutes.

Drain the lentils, reserving 2½ C. of the cooking liquid.

Meanwhile, in another large pan, heat the oil over medium heat and sauté the onion for about 2-3 minutes.

Add in the garlic and sauté for about 1 minute.

Add the tomatoes and cook for about 5 minutes.

Stir in the curry powder and spices and cook for about 1 minute.

Add the carrots, potatoes, pumpkin, cooked lentils and reserved cooking liquid and bring to a gentle boil.

Reduce the heat to medium-low and simmer, covered for about 40-45 minutes or until desired doneness of the vegetables.

Stir in the apple and spinach and simmer for about 15 minutes.

Stir in the salt and black pepper and remove from the heat.

Serve hot.

Nutrition:

Calories per serving: 263; Carbohydrates: 47g; Protein: 14.7g; Fat: 2.9g; Sugar: 9.7g; Sodium: 53mg; Fiber: 20g

181.   Omega-3 Rich Dinner Meal

Preparation Time: 15 minutes

Cooking Time: 40 minutes

Servings: 4

Ingredients:

For Lentils:

½ lb. French green lentils

2 tbsp. extra-virgin olive oil

2 C. yellow onions, chopped

2 C. scallions, chopped

1 tsp. fresh parsley, chopped

Salt and freshly ground black pepper, to taste

1 tbsp. garlic, minced

1½ C. carrots, peeled and chopped

1½ C. celery stalks, chopped

1 large tomato, peeled, seeded and crushed finely

1½ C. chicken bone broth

2 tbsp. balsamic vinegar

For Salmon:

2 (8-oz.) skinless salmon fillets

2 tbsp. extra-virgin olive oil

Salt and freshly ground black pepper, to taste

Directions:

Ina heat-proof bowl, soak the lentils in boiling water for 15 minutes.

Drain the lentils completely.

In a Dutch oven, heat the oil in over medium heat and cook the onions, scallions, parsley, salt and black pepper for about 10 minutes, stirring frequently.

Add the garlic and cook for about 2 more minutes.

Add the drained lentils, carrots, celery, crushed tomato and broth and bring to a boil.

Reduce the heat to low and simmer, covered for about 20-25 minutes.

Stir in the vinegar, salt and black pepper and remove from the heat.

Meanwhile, for salmon: preheat your oven to 450 degrees F.

Rub the salmon fillets with oil and then, season with salt and black pepper generously.

Heat an oven-proof sauté pan over medium heat and cook the salmon fillets for about 2minutes, without stirring.

Flip the fillets and immediately transfer the pan into the oven.

Bake for about 5-7 minutes or until desired doneness of salmon.

Remove from the oven and place the salmon fillets onto a cutting board.

Cut each fillet into 2 portions.

Divide the lentil mixture onto serving plates and top each with 1 salmon fillet.

Serve hot.

Nutrition:

Calories per serving: 707; Carbohydrates: 50.2g; Protein: 16.1g; Fat: 29.8g;

Sugar: 7.9g; Sodium: 496mg; Fiber: 16.2g

182.   <u>Weekend Dinner Casserole</u>

Preparation Time: 20 minutes

Cooking Time: 1 hour

Servings: 6

Ingredients:

2½ C. water, divided

1 C. red lentils

½ C. wild rice

1 tsp. olive oil

1 small onion, chopped

3 garlic cloves, minced

1/3 C. zucchini, peeled, seeded and chopped

1/3 C. carrot, peeled and chopped

1/3 C. celery stalk, chopped

1 large tomato, peeled, seeded and chopped

8 oz. tomato sauce

1 tsp. ground cumin

1 tsp. dried oregano, crushed

1 tsp. dried basil, crushed

Salt and freshly ground black pepper, to taste

Directions:

In a pan, add 1 C. of the water and rice over medium-high heat and bring to a rolling boil.

Reduce the heat to low and simmer, covered for about 20 minutes.

Meanwhile, in another pan, add the remaining water and lentils over medium heat and bring to a rolling boil.

Reduce the heat to low and simmer, covered for about 15 minutes.

Transfer the cooked rice and lentils into a casserole dish and set aside.

Preheat your oven to 350 degrees F.

Heat the oil in a large skillet over medium heat and sauté the onion and garlic for about 4-5 minutes.

Add the zucchini, carrot, celery, tomato and tomato paste and cook for about 4-5 minutes.

Stir in the cumin, herbs, salt and black pepper and remove from the heat.

Transfer the vegetable mixture into the casserole dish with rice and lentils and stir to combine.

Bake for about 30 minutes.

Remove from the heat and set aside for about 5 minutes.

Cut into equal-sized 6 pieces and serve.

Nutrition:

Calories per serving: 192; Carbohydrates: 34.5g; Protein: 11.3g; Fat: 1.5g; Sugar: 3.9g; Sodium: 239mg; Fiber: 12g

183.   Family Dinner Pilaf

Preparation Time: 15 minutes

Cooking Time: 1 hour

Servings: 4

Ingredients:

2 tbsp. olive oil

2 garlic cloves, minced

2 C. fresh mushrooms, sliced

1¼ C. brown rice, rinsed

2 C. homemade vegetable broth

Salt and freshly ground black pepper, to taste

1 red bell pepper, seeded and chopped

4 scallions, chopped

1 (16-oz.) can red kidney beans, drained and rinsed

2 tbsp. fresh parsley, chopped

Directions:

In a large pan, heat the oil over medium heat and sauté the onion for about 4-5 minutes.

Add the garlic and mushrooms and cook about 5-6 minutes.

Stir in the rice and cook for about 1-2 minutes, stirring continuously.

Stir in the broth, salt and black pepper and bring to a boil.

Reduce the heat to low and simmer, covered for about 35 minutes, stirring occasionally.

Add in the bell pepper and beans and cook for about 5-10 minutes or until all the liquid is absorbed.

Serve hot with the garnishing of parsley.

Nutrition:

Calories per serving: 463; Carbohydrates: 76.7g; Protein: 18.5g; Fat: 10.1g; Sugar: 3.2g; Sodium: 431mg; Fiber: 11.6g

184.   Meat-Free Bolognese Pasta

Preparation Time: 20 minutes

Cooking Time: 2 hours

Servings: 5

Ingredients:

For Bolognese Sauce:

5 tbsp. olive oil, divided

3 celery stalks, chopped finely

1 medium carrot, peeled and chopped finely

1 medium onion, chopped finely

1 C. quinoa, rinsed

3 C. fresh mushrooms, chopped

4 garlic cloves, chopped

¾ tsp. dried oregano

½ tsp. dried thyme

¼ tsp. dried rosemary

¼ tsp. dried sage

1/8 tsp. red pepper flakes

1½ C. homemade vegetable broth

2 cups tomatoes, peeled, seeded and crushed finely

½-1 C. water

1 tbsp. balsamic vinegar

4 bay leaves

2 tbsp. nutritional yeast

¼ C. oat milk

Salt and freshly ground black pepper, to taste

¼ C. fresh basil leaves

For Pasta:

¾ lb. whole-wheat pasta (of your choice)

Directions:

Preheat your oven to 300 degrees F.

In a large Dutch oven, heat 3 tbsp. of the olive oil over medium heat and cook the celery, carrots and onion for about 10 minutes, stirring frequently.

Stir in the quinoa and cook for about 3 minutes.

Add the remaining oil and mushrooms and stir to combine.

Increase the heat to medium-high and cook for about 5 minutes.

Add the garlic, dried herbs and red pepper flakes and cook for about 1-2 minutes.

Add the broth and cook for about 5 minutes.

Add the tomatoes, water, vinegar and bay leaves and bring to a boil.

Remove the Dutch oven from heat and transfer into the oven.

Bake, uncovered for about 1½ hours, stirring once after 1 hour.

Meanwhile, in a pan of the lightly salted boiling water, cook the pasta for about 8-10 minutes or according to package's instructions.

Drin the pasta well.

Remove the Dutch oven from oven and stir in the nutritional yeast and oat milk.

Divide the pasta onto serving plates and top with Bolognese sauce.

Garnish with basil leaves and serve.

Nutrition:

Calories per serving: 510; Carbohydrates: 71g; Protein: 17.1g; Fat: 18.3g; Sugar: 5.9g; Sodium: 241mg; Fiber: 6.5g

185.   Pasta with Escarole, Beans and Turkey

Preparation Time: 20 mins.

Cooking Time: 16mins.

Servings: 4

Ingredients:

whole-wheat bowtie pasta (3/4 pound)

olive oil (1 tbs)

onion (1/2 medium, chopped)

cloves garlic (3, minced)

turkey (6 oz, ground)

head escarole (1 medium, rinsed, drained and chopped)

cannellini beans (1(14oz) can, drained and rinsed)

chicken broth (1 1/2 cups)

rosemary (1 tbs, chopped)

salt (1/2 tsp)

Parmesan cheese (1/4 cup, grated)

Directions:

Bring a salted water to boil in a pot. Add the pasta and follow the cooking instruction on the package.

Drain. In a large non-stick pan, heat olive oil over medium heat.

Add onion and cook until softened, add garlic and turkey and cook until it browns, about 5 minutes.

Add the escarole and cook it for 4 minutes. Add the beans, 1 cup of turkey stock, rosemary, and salt.

Simmer until the mixture is slightly thickened. Add the pasta and toss well, thin the sauce with the additional 1/2 cup stock if needed.

Top with parmesan cheese. Serve.

Nutrition:

289 calories, 6 g fat,36 g carbs, 16 g fiber, 24 g protein

186.   Rice Bowl with Shrimp and Peas

Preparation Time: 15 mins.

Cooking Time: 48 mins.

Servings: 4

Ingredients:

long-grain brown rice (1 cup)

soy sauce (1/4 cup)

fresh lemon juice (1/4 cup)

rice vinegar (2 tbs)

honey (2 tbs)

olive oil (1 tbs)

shrimp (1 lb, medium, cleaned, peeled, deveined)

snow peas (8 oz, thawed if frozen, cut in halves)

piece fresh ginger (1 (1-inch long) shredded)

Hass avocado (1, chopped)

Directions:

Boil 2 cups of water in a saucepan. Add the rice and cover and turn the heat down to simmer.

Cook the rice for about 35-45 minutes. In a bowl, fully combine soy sauce, lemon juice, honey, and vinegar.

Set your olive oil to get hot on medium heat in a non-stick pan.

Add in your shrimp, ginger and peas then cook for about 3 minutes (or until shrimp becomes pink).

Transfer rice to serving bowls, then top with avocado and shrimp mixture. Serve the sauce on the side.

Nutrition:

143 calories, 4 g fat, 19g carbs, 2 g fiber, 7 g protein

187.   Roasted Chicken and Vegetables

Preparation Time: 15 mins.

Cooking Time: 55 mins.

Servings: 4

Ingredients:

Roma tomatoes (6, seedless, quartered)

Zucchini (3 medium, chopped coarsely)

Potatoes (2 large, unpeeled, quartered)

olive oil (3 tbs, divided)

salt (3/4 tsp, divided)

cloves garlic (4, finely minced)

fresh rosemary (1 tbs, chopped)

fresh thyme (1 tbs, leaves taken off sprig)

lemon zest (1 tsp)

lemon juice (1 tbs)

chicken breast halves (4, skinless)

Directions:

Preheat oven to 375F degrees. Put tomatoes, zucchini and potatoes in a roasting pan, and toss with 2 tbs of oil and 1/4 tsp salt.

Combine lemon zest, thyme, rosemary, garlic, oil, salt and lemon juice. Pour this mixture over chicken.

Place chicken in pan with vegetables. Bake in oven for 30 minutes.

Stir chicken and vegetables and bake another 25 minutes, or until chicken is cooked through and vegetables are tender.

Nutrition:

147 calories, 11 g fat, 13g carbs, 3 g fiber, 2 g protein

188. Shrimp and Black Bean Nachos

Preparation Time: 25 mins.

Cooking Time: 0 mins.

Servings: 4

Ingredients:

Cilantro (3/4 cup, fresh chopped)

red onion (1/2 cup, diced)

lime juice (2 tbs)

olive oil (1 tbs)

Worcestershire sauce (1 tsp)

salt (1/2 tsp)

shrimp (3/4 lb medium, peeled, cooked, and chopped)

tomatoes (2 cups, seeded, diced)

avocado (1/2 cup, diced)

black bean (1 (15 oz) can, rinsed and drained)

ground cumin (1/2 tsp)

baked tortilla chips (4 cup)

Directions:

In a bowl combine cilantro, onion, lime juice, oil, Worcestershire sauce, shrimp and salt. Cover and refrigerate for 30 minutes.

Add tomato and avocado; stir well. Place the cumin and beans in a food processor, and process until smooth.

Spread 1-teaspoon black-bean mixture on each chip. Top with 1-tablespoon shrimp mixture. Serve.

Nutrition:

172 calories, 14 g fat, 12 g carbs, 5 g fiber, 4 g protein

189.   Southwestern Chicken Pitas

Preparation Time: 15 mins.

Cooking Time: 0 mins.

Servings: 6

Ingredients:

black beans (1 (15 oz) can, drained, rinsed)

red bell pepper (1/2 cup, chopped, seeded)

fresh lime juice (3 tbs)

fresh cilantro leaves (2 tbs, minced)

canola oil (2 tbs)

chicken breasts (4, boneless, halved, skinless)

round whole wheat pita bread (4)

low-fat provolone cheese (6 slices, cut in halves)

Directions:

In a bowl, combine beans, bell pepper, lime juice, and cilantro. Set aside. In a pan, heat up the oil over medium heat.

Cook chicken in pan until golden brown. Set aside for 10 without cutting. Warm pita bread in oven.

Cut chicken into slices. Place half a slice of cheese in center of one pita bread.

Top off the sandwich with bean mixture the chicken breast slices. Roll up tightly. Cut in half and serve.

Nutrition:

345 calories, 12 g fat, 22 g carbs, 5 g fiber, 35 g protein

190.   Spaghetti with Zucchini

Preparation Time: 10 mins.

Cooking Time: 12 mins.

Servings: 4

Ingredients:

whole wheat spaghetti (1 lb)

zucchini (2 medium, grated, water, squeezed out)

butter (2 tbs)

olive oil (1 tbs)

cloves garlic (2, minced)

Parmesan cheese (1/2 cup, freshly grated)

Directions:

Bring a salted water to boil in a pot. Add pasta and cook until it is al dente or follow the instructions on the package.

While pasta cooks, in a large non-stick pan, heat the oil and butter together. Add in the zucchini and allow cook for 3 minutes.

Add in your garlic and continue to cook for another minute, stirring constantly. Add in a half of your parmesan cheese.

Transfer past to a serving bowl. Add your zucchini mixture. Toss then garnish with remaining parmesan cheese. Enjoy!

Nutrition:

156 calories, 11 g fat, 11 g carbs, 2 g fiber, 5 g protein

191.   Summer Spaghetti

Preparation Time: 15 mins.

Cooking Time: 8 mins.

Servings: 4

Ingredients:

whole wheat spaghetti (1 lb)

olive oil (1/4 cup)

shallot (1, minced)

cloves garlic (2, minced)

zucchini (1 medium, chopped)

summer squash (1 medium, chopped)

green beans (1/2 lb, ends cut)

basil (1/4 cup, coarsely chopped)

salt (1/2 tsp)

lemon (1/2 medium, juiced)

unsalted butter (2 tbs, room temperature)

freshly grated lemon peel

Directions:

Bring a salted water to boil in a pot. Add pasta and cook until it is al dente or follow the instructions on the package.

Heat up the oil over medium heat in a large pan. Add in your garlic and shallot, then stir frequently until fragrant (about 2 minutes).

Add the zucchini, squash, green beans, and basil. Continue to cook, stir occasionally, until all vegetables are tender.

Season vegetables with salt and lemon juice. In a large shallow pasta bowl, immediately place the sautéed vegetables with all their juices.

Add the butter and linguine, toss to mix well and serve immediately.

Nutrition:

548 calories, 57 g fat, 14 g carbs, 3 g fiber, 3 g protein

192.   Pink Salmon Cakes & Potatoes

Preparation Time: 20 mins.

Cooking Time: 16 mins.

Servings: 4

Ingredients:

For Pink salmon Cakes:

canola oil (3 tbs)

pink salmon fish (2 (6 oz) cans, drained)

egg (1, beaten)

green onions (2 tablespoons, diced)

mayonnaise (1/4 cup, non-fat)

whole wheat bread (1/2 cup, cut into small pieces)

Lemon juice, optional

For Smashed Potatoes:

Potatoes (2 large, unpeeled, chopped)

salt (2 tsp)

low fat milk (1/2 cup)

unsalted butter (3 tablespoons)

Directions:

Cook potatoes in a small saucepan until tender. Drain.

Place potatoes back in pan. Heat the butter and milk in microwave until hot.

Roughly smash the potatoes with a potato smasher while adding hot liquid until combined and set aside.

Combine egg, pink salmon, lemon juice, green onions, mayonnaise, breadcrumbs, and egg in a bowl.

Form into patties. Allow to refrigerate and become firm for 10 minutes.

Heat oil over medium heat, cook patties until golden brown, about 2 minutes on each side. Serve with potatoes.

Nutrition:

432 calories, 34 g fat, 29 g carbs, 2 g fiber, 6 g protein

193.   Turkey and Barley Casserole

Preparation Time: 15 mins.

Cooking Time: 1 hr. 10 mins.

Servings: 4

Ingredients:

ground turkey (3/4 lb)

salt (1/2 tsp)

onion (1, chopped finely)

carrots (2, chopped)

stalks celery (2, chopped)

green bell pepper (1, seeded and chopped)

button mushrooms (12, quartered)

chicken stock (2 1/2 cups)

barley (1 cup)

poultry seasoning (1 tsp)

bay leaf (1)

Directions:

Preheat oven to 375F degrees. Over medium heat, cook ground turkey with salt until browned, about 5 minutes, in a pan.

Add green peppers, celery, carrots and onions. Cook until tender, about 5 minutes.

Add bay leaf, poultry seasoning, barley, stock and mushrooms.

Mix together and place the mixture in a baking dish. Cover and bake in the preheated oven for 1 hour. Serve.

Nutrition:

361 calories, 11 g fat, 42 g carbs, 10 g fiber, 30 g protein

Dessert

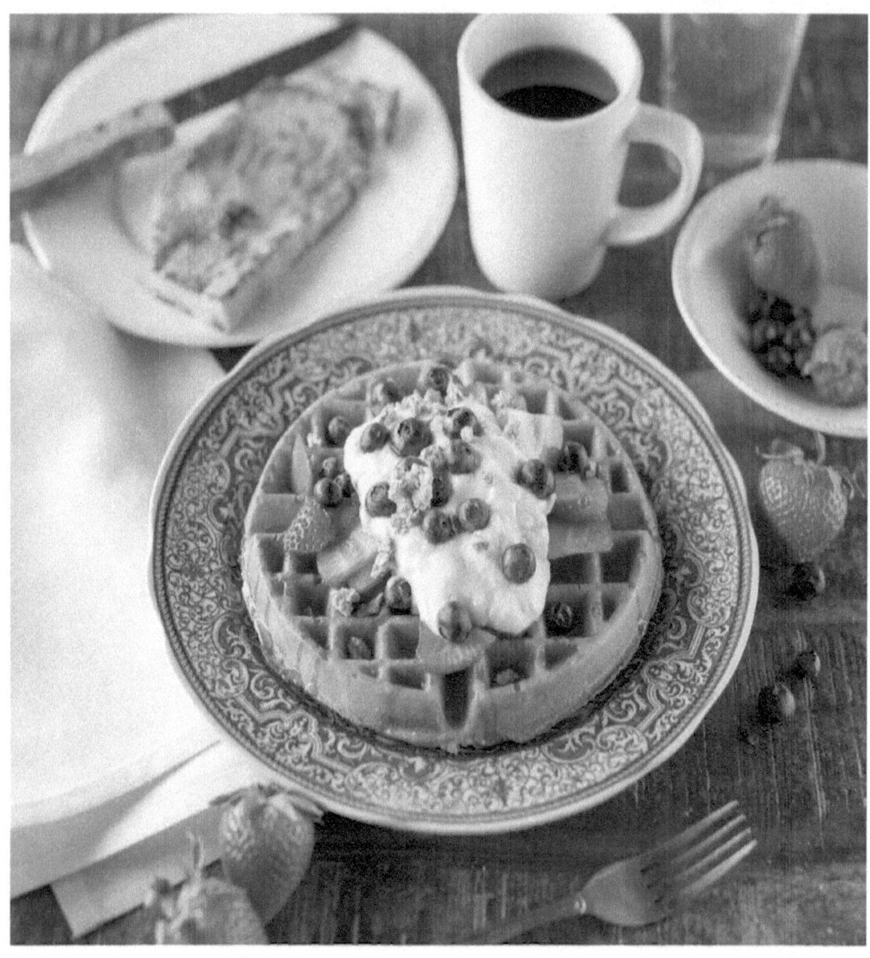

194. <u>Baked Pears with Homemade Granola</u>

Preparation Time: 10 minutes

Cooking Time: 40 minutes

Servings: 8

Ingredients:

FOR THE GRANOLA

1 cup rolled oats

¼ cup almonds

1 tablespoon chia seeds

1 tablespoon hemp seeds

1 tablespoon pumpkin or sunflower seeds

½ teaspoon ground cinnamon

Pinch salt

1 tablespoon coconut oil, melted

2 teaspoons maple syrup

¼ teaspoon vanilla extract

FOR THE PEARS

4 Anjou pears

½ cup maple syrup

1 teaspoon vanilla extract

½ teaspoon ground cinnamon

To make the granola

Directions:

Preheat the oven to 375°F. Line a baking sheet with parchment paper.

In a large bowl, mix together the oats, almonds, chia seeds, hemp seeds, pumpkin seeds, cinnamon, and salt.

In a small bowl, mix together the coconut oil, maple syrup, and vanilla. Drizzle the mixture over the oat mixture and stir to combine.

Spread the oat mixture out onto the prepared baking sheet. Bake for 10 minutes and stir well. Continue to bake for another 10 minutes. Let cool on a wire rack.

To make the pears

Line the baking sheet with another sheet of parchment paper.

Cut the pears in half lengthwise. Cut a very small slice off the rounded side of each half, which will help the pears sit flat. Using a melon baller or a spoon, scoop out the core and seeds. Place the pear halves on the prepared baking sheet.

Spoon the granola into the pears.

In a small bowl, whisk together the maple syrup and vanilla and drizzle it over the pears. Sprinkle the cinnamon over the pear halves.

Bake for 15 to 20 minutes, or until the pears are cooked through and tender. Serve immediately.

Nutrition: Calories: 196; Fat: 2g; Carbohydrates: 34g; Fiber: 5g; Protein: 4g; Sodium: 5mg; Vitamin B12: 0%; Iron: 9%

195. Avocado Chia Pudding Four Ways

Preparation Time: 10 minutes

Cooking Time: 0 minutes

Servings: 4

Ingredients:

FOR THE PUDDING BASE

2 cups milk of choice

½ avocado, mashed

½ cup chia seeds

3 tablespoons honey, plus more as needed

½ teaspoon vanilla extract

FLAVOR OPTIONS

CHOCOLATE

¼ cup unsweetened cocoa powder

PUMPKIN SPICE

½ cup pumpkin puree

1 teaspoon ground cinnamon

¼ teaspoon ground ginger

Pinch ground cloves

APPLE PIE

½ cup applesauce

1 teaspoon ground cinnamon

¼ teaspoon ground ginger

Pinch ground cloves

BERRY

½ cup berries of choice

Directions:

Put the milk, avocado, chia seeds, honey, and vanilla in a food processor or a blender and puree until smooth. Taste, and add more honey, if desired.

Add the ingredients for your choice of flavors and puree.

Pour the mixture into bowls or mason jars, cover, and refrigerate for at least 2 hours.

Nutrition: Calories: 257; Fat: 11g; Carbohydrates: 31g; Fiber: 12g; Protein: 11g; Sodium: 56mg; Vitamin B12: 9%; Iron: 13%

196.   Dark Chocolate Brownies

Preparation Time: 10 minutes

Cooking Time: 35 minutes

Servings: Makes 9 brownies

Ingredients:

¾ cup dark chocolate chips

8 tablespoons (1 stick) butter or margarine

½ (15½-ounce) can black beans, drained and rinsed

½ cup sugar

2 large eggs

2 teaspoons vanilla extract

1¾ cups whole-wheat flour

2 tablespoons unsweetened dark cocoa powder

Pinch salt

Directions:

Preheat the oven to 350°F. Line a 9-by-9-inch square baking pan with aluminum foil or parchment paper and grease well. Set aside.

In a microwave-safe bowl, melt the chocolate chips and butter in the microwave in 20-second intervals, stirring occasionally, until smooth. Let cool.

In a blender, puree the beans, adding water 1 teaspoon at a time, until smooth. Set aside.

Add the sugar to the cooled chocolate and whisk to combine. Whisk in the eggs, one at a time. Add the vanilla and pureed black beans and stir to combine.

Gradually mix in the flour, cocoa powder, and salt until well combined.

Pour the batter into the prepared pan, spreading it evenly. Bake for 30 to 35 minutes, or until a toothpick inserted into the middle comes clean. Let cool completely in the pan on a wire rack. Remove the brownies from the pan by lifting the foil. Cut into 9 bars.

Let stand at room temperature for at least 30 minutes before serving.

Store the brownies wrapped in plastic wrap at room temperature for up to 2 days or in the refrigerator for up to 4 months.

Nutrition: Calories: 301; Fat: 13g; Carbohydrates: 42g; Fiber: 6g; Protein: 6g; Sodium: 106mg; Vitamin B12: 2%; Iron: 12%

197. Chocolate Chip Protein Bites

Preparation Time: 10 minutes

Cooking Time: ½ cup Rice Krispies

Servings: Makes 10 protein bites

Ingredients:

½ cup natural nut butter

½ cup rolled oats

1/3 cup ground flaxseed

¼ cup honey or maple syrup

2 tablespoons hemp seeds

1 tablespoon chia seeds

1 tablespoon chocolate chips

1 teaspoon vanilla extract

½ teaspoon ground cinnamon

Directions:

In a large bowl, mix together the Rice Krispies, nut butter, oats, flaxseed, honey, hemp seeds, chia seeds, chocolate chips, vanilla, and cinnamon until well combined.

Using your hands, roll the mixture into 10 balls. If the mixture is really sticky, wear food-safe plastic gloves to roll them.

Store the balls in an airtight container in the freezer for up to 3 months.

Nutrition: Calories: 166; Fat: 10g; Carbohydrates: 16g; Fiber: 3g; Protein: 5g; Sodium: 70mg; Vitamin B12: 3%; Iron: 7%

198.   Oat Bars with Raspberry Chia Jam

Preparation Time: 15 minutes

Cooking Time: 25 minutes

Servings: Makes 9 bars

Ingredients:

FOR THE JAM

1 cup frozen raspberries

2 tablespoons chia seeds

1 tablespoon honey

1 teaspoon vanilla extract

FOR THE OAT BARS

2 cups whole-wheat flour

1 1/3 cups rolled oats

1 cup brown sugar

1 cup (2 sticks) butter or margarine, at room temperature

2 teaspoons ground cinnamon

1 teaspoon vanilla extract

To make the jam

Directions:

In a microwave-safe bowl, heat the raspberries in the microwave, in 1-minute intervals, until soft.

Add the chia seeds, honey, and vanilla and let sit until thickened, about 5 minutes.

To make the oat bars

Preheat the oven to 350°F. Grease an 8-by-8-inch baking dish. Set aside.

In a large bowl, mix together the flour, oats, brown sugar, butter, cinnamon, and vanilla.

Press about two-thirds of the mixture into the prepared baking dish. Using a spoon, spread the chia jam over the oat mixture, leaving a ½-inch space around the edges to prevent the jam from burning when it's baked.

Sprinkle the remaining oat mixture over the jam.

Bake for 20 to 25 minutes, or until the bars are golden brown. Let cool completely on a wire rack.

Once cooled, cut into 9 bars and serve.

Helpful Hint: These taste really great topped with a scoop of vanilla ice cream. Or serve them for breakfast with a spoonful of plain or vanilla Greek yogurt.

Nutrition: Calories: 407; Fat: 22g; Carbohydrates: 51g; Fiber: 6g; Protein: 6g; Sodium: 152mg; Vitamin B12: 1%; Iron: 14%

199. Almond-Orange Cranberry Loaf

Preparation Time: 10 minutes

Cooking Time: 55 minutes

Servings: Makes 1 loaf (12 servings)

Ingredients:

2 cups whole-wheat flour

1 teaspoon ground cinnamon

1 teaspoon baking powder

½ teaspoon baking soda

1/3 cup sugar

4 tablespoons (½ stick) butter or margarine, at room temperature

2 large eggs

1 cup freshly squeezed orange juice

1 cup dried unsweetened cranberries

¾ cup sliced almonds

2 tablespoons chia seeds

1 teaspoon orange zest

Directions:

Preheat the oven to 350°F. Grease a 5-by-9-inch loaf pan and set aside.

In a large bowl, combine the flour, cinnamon, baking powder, and baking soda. Set aside.

In a separate bowl, whisk together the sugar and butter until light and fluffy. Add the eggs one at a time, whisking well to incorporate. Add the orange juice and whisk until well mixed.

Form a well in the center of the dry ingredients. Add the sugar mixture and fold in using a rubber spatula. Add the cranberries, almonds, chia, and orange zest and fold into the batter. Be careful not to overmix, or the loaf will be tough.

Pour the batter into the prepared loaf pan and spread out evenly. Bake for 50 to 55 minutes, or until a toothpick inserted into the center comes out clean.

Let cool in the pan on a wire rack for 10 minutes. Remove the loaf from the pan and cool completely before serving.

Nutrition: Calories: 187; Fat: 6g; Carbohydrates: 29g; Fiber: 3g; Protein: 4g; Sodium: 229mg; Vitamin B12: 2%; Iron: 8%

200.   Gingerbread Pancakes

Preparation Time: 15 minutes

Cooking Time: 25 minutes

Servings: 4

Ingredients:

½ cup whole-wheat flour

¼ cup sugar

1½ teaspoons baking powder

½ teaspoon baking soda

½ teaspoon salt

1 cup canned lentils, rinsed

2 large eggs

¼ cup molasses

¼ cup milk of choice

3 tablespoons canola oil

1 teaspoon ground ginger

1 teaspoon ground cinnamon

½ teaspoon ground cloves

1 teaspoon vegetable oil or cooking spray

Directions:

In a medium bowl, sift together the flour, sugar, baking powder, baking soda, and salt. Set aside.

Place the lentils in a blender or food processor and puree until completely smooth. Add water 1 tablespoon at a time to thin enough to puree.

In a separate large bowl, whisk together the eggs, molasses, milk, canola oil, ginger, cinnamon, and cloves.

Mix the flour mixture into the lentil mixture and stir until smooth.

Set a large sauté pan or skillet over medium heat. Lightly grease with the vegetable oil. Spoon ¼ cup of batter into the skillet and cook until bubbles start to form around the edges, 2 to 3 minutes. Flip and cook until golden brown, another 2 to 3 minutes. Serve with desired toppings.

Store leftovers in the refrigerator for up to 5 days or in the freezer for up to 4 months. To reheat, heat in the microwave until hot.

Nutrition: Calories: 365; Fat: 15g; Carbohydrates: 49g; Fiber: 6g; Protein: 10g; Sodium: 683mg; Vitamin B12: 5%; Iron: 23%

Chapter 7. 21 Day Meal Plan

Days	Breakfast	Lunch	Snack	Dinner	Dessert
7 Day Phase 1					
1	Blueberry Green Tea	Slow Cooker Pork Bone Broth	3-Ingredient Sugar Free Gelatin	Asian Inspired Wonton Broth	Tropical Fruit Punch
2	Raspberry Lemonade Ice Pops	Homemade Chicken Stock	Strawberry Gummies	Oxtail Bone Broth	Pineapple Ice Cubes
3	Pineapple Mint Juice	Best Homemade Broth	Fruity Jell-O Stars	Beef Bone Broth	Banana Ice Cubes
4	Homemade Banana Apple Juice	Healing Broth	Plum and Nectarine Gelatin Pudding	Ginger, Mushroom & Cauliflower Broth	Frozen Strawberry-Peach Pops
5	Sweet Detox Juice	Brain Healthy Broth	Homemade Lemon Gelatin	Pork Stock	Melon Basil Moscow Mule Popsicles
6	Carrot Orange Juice	Minerals Rich Broth	Sour Blueberry Gummies	Indian Inspired Vegetable stock	Strawberry Popsicles
7	Strawberry Apple Juice	Holiday Favorite Gelatin	Sugar – Free Cinnamon Jelly	Clear Pumpkin Broth	Basil Watermelon Popsicles
7 Day Phase 2					

8	Spinach Frittata	Family Favorite Scramble	Almond Peanut Butter Fudge	Flavorful Shrimp Kabobs	Banana Cocoa Cream
9	Pear Pancakes	Garden Veggies Quiche	Quick Cocoa Mousse	Pan-Seared Scallops	Homemade Pumpkin Pie
10	Apple Oatmeal	Classic Zucchini Bread	Cinnamon Pear Chips	Helth Conscious People's Salad	Chocolate Pear Cream
11	Zucchini Omelet	Light Veggie Salad	Chocolate Yogurt Cream & Roasted Bananas	Italian Pasta Soup	Zero Sugar Pumpkin Pie
12	Coconut Chia Seed Pudding	Citrus Glazed Carrots	Coconut Celery Smoothie	Zero-Fiber Chicken Dish	Orange Curd
13	Breakfast Cereal	Braised Asparagus	Apple Spinach Smoothie	Colorful Chicken Dinner	Instant Pot Pear Crumble
14	Strawberry Cashew Chia Pudding	Gluten-Free Curry	Cinnamon Pear Chips	Lemony Salmon	Sweet Potato Cream Pie

7 Day Phase 3

15	Healthier Breakfast Juice	South Western Salad	Ricotta & Cannellini Salad	Thanksgiving Dinner Chili	Baked Pears with Homemade Granola
16	Frilling Breakfast	Eye-Catching	String bean	Beans Trio Chili	Avocado Chia

	Smoothie	Sweet Potato Boats	Potato Salad		Pudding Four Ways
17	Quickest Breakfast Porridge	Armenian Style Chickpeas	Cucumber Peach Salad	Weekend Dinner Casserole	Dark Chocolate Brownies
18	Halloween Morning Oatmeal	One-Pot Dinner Soup	Strawberry & Apple Salad	Pasta with Escarole, Beans and Turkey	Chocolate Chip Protein Bites
19	Authentic Bulgur Porridge	Chicken and Quinoa Pita	Bean and Couscous Salad	Shrimp and Black Bean Nachos	Oat Bars with Raspberry Chia Jam
20	Savory Crepes	Chicken Lettuce Wraps	Almond Salad	Summer Spaghetti	Almond-Orange Cranberry Loaf
21	Summer Treat Salad	Ham, Bean and Cabbage Stew	Nutty Green Salad	Pink Salmon Cakes & Potatoes	Gingerbread Pancakes

Conclusion

The term diverticulosis and diverticulitis are often confused with each other. People confuse themselves to have diverticulitis when all they have is common diverticulosis. Diverticulosis is a common infection while diverticulitis is a more serious condition and is caused due to acute inflammation of the bowel wall. It is not easy to cure diverticulitis and it often calls for treatment through antibiotics.

In extreme situations, patient may also be required to undergo surgery and has to be kept under prolonged medical supervision. Diverticulosis on the other hand is the condition where people have large intestinal pockets known as diverticula. This condition is sufficiently common and does pose serious consequences. It can be treated with normal dietary and lifestyle changes.

The convenient way to differentiate between the two terms is to remember the term 'itis'. Any disease ending with this term generally represents some kind of inflammation. The common medical precaution is to minimize the chances of the inflammation to burst. In case it bursts, it can be severely life threatening.

Diverticulitis is generally observed in the colon or large bowel as holes or multiple pockets. They are named as holes but have a very thin lining that prevents the stool and bacteria to pass out to the wall of the colon. The lining is excessively thin and any unwanted pressure on it causes the diverticulum to break. The breakage of this lining is responsible for the spread of bacteria and stool onto the wall of the colon thus infecting it severely. Such breakage may also lead to walled off infection that gets filled with bacteria and pus. This formation is known as abscess. The infection does not remain confined to the colon wall but is likely to spread to the other adjacent organs like ovaries, bladder, uterus etc. The bladder often suffers a condition of holes formation known as fistula. Other commonly reported situation is the passing of air while the patient urinates. Curing the abscess is a very difficult and complicated since other organs are involved and are prone to damage.

Diverticulosis has common occurrence and no significant symptoms. It is known to adopt progression and cannot be cured completely. The only way to control it is early detection and adopting preventive measures. Diverticulosis is presence of pockets in the colon which are not harmful. The real problem is the high pressured zones created due to thickened muscles known as mychosis. This thickening generates in the sigmoid colon in the left lower abdomen. This condition may cause austere narrowing and muscle buildup leading to muscle contractions. These contractions cause excruciating pain. They may also lead to extreme high pressures that can pressurize the colon walls, causing them to burst and spread infection in and around the colon wall. This is the condition which in severe cases leads to formation of diverticulitis. A high fiber diet and plentiful of liquid intake are the only ways through which diverticulosis can be kept under check.